# Caffeine
# for Sports
# Performance

Louise Burke, PhD
Ben Desbrow, PhD
Lawrence Spriet, PhD

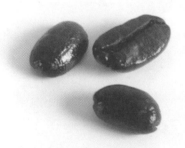

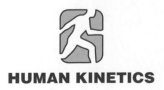

**HUMAN KINETICS**

**Library of Congress Cataloging-in-Publication Data**

Burke, Louise, 1959-
   Caffeine for sports performance / Louise Burke, Ben Desbrow, and Lawrence Spriet.
      pages cm
   Includes bibliographical references and index.
   1. Athletes--Nutrition. 2. Athletes--Health and hygiene. 3. Caffeine--Health aspects. I. Title.
   TX361.A8B88 2013
   613.8'4--dc23

                                 2012049486

ISBN-10: 0-7360-9511-X (print)
ISBN-13: 978-0-7360-9511-2 (print)

**Acquisitions Editor:** Tom Heine; **Developmental Editor:** Jacqueline Eaton Blakley; **Assistant Editor:** Anne Rumery; **Copyeditor:** Alisha Jeddeloh; **Indexer:** Andrea Hepner; **Permissions Manager:** Martha Gullo; **Graphic Designer:** Joe Buck; **Graphic Artist:** Tara Welsch; **Cover Designer:** Keith Blomberg; **Photograph (cover and interior):** Neil Bernstein; **Art Manager:** Kelly Hendren; **Associate Art Manager:** Alan L. Wilborn; **Illustrations:** © Human Kinetics, unless otherwise noted; **Printer:** Versa Press

Printed in the United States of America        10   9   8   7   6   5   4   3   2   1

The paper in this book is certified under a sustainable forestry program.

**Human Kinetics**
Website: www.HumanKinetics.com

*United States:* Human Kinetics
P.O. Box 5076
Champaign, IL 61825-5076
800-747-4457
e-mail: humank@hkusa.com

*Canada:* Human Kinetics
475 Devonshire Road Unit 100
Windsor, ON N8Y 2L5
800-465-7301 (in Canada only)
e-mail: info@hkcanada.com

*Europe:* Human Kinetics
107 Bradford Road
Stanningley
Leeds LS28 6AT, United Kingdom
+44 (0) 113 255 5665
e-mail: hk@hkeurope.com

*Australia:* Human Kinetics
57A Price Avenue
Lower Mitcham, South Australia 5062
08 8372 0999
e-mail: info@hkaustralia.com

*New Zealand:* Human Kinetics
P.O. Box 80
Torrens Park, South Australia 5062
0800 222 062
e-mail: info@hknewzealand.com

E5172

For Anne, Andrew, Stephanie, and Sarah—you keep me high on life, and then some!

—Lawrence


For Jane, Jemima, and Ella—my three strongest addictions.

—Ben


For John and Jack, the boys who give me wings, and in honor of the Coke habit of the older one and the caffeine-free energy of the younger. Things go better with you two around me.

—Louise

# Contents

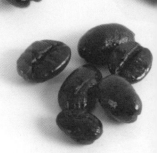

# Preface

Professor Ron Maughan, a world-renowned sport nutrition expert, often talks about his three laws of dietary supplements and sports performance:

1. If a supplement works, it's probably illegal (for use in sport).
2. If a supplement is legal, it probably doesn't work.
3. There may be exceptions.

This book is about one of the exceptions.

Caffeine is a fascinating substance that has become entrenched in our everyday lives. Around the world, most adults consume it on a daily basis in a variety of forms. Many people consider their caffeine habits to be an important social activity or linked to their quality of life or dietary enjoyment. In fact, the underlying reason for caffeine intake is usually performance. Whether we realize it or not, most of us consume caffeine to help us get through the day feeling better, having more energy, or being able to achieve our daily tasks more effectively. Most people seem to work out a way to get the best out of the ability of caffeine to assist with these goals. At times, however, some of us get it wrong and suffer from side effects or poor use outcomes. We have had centuries of experience with caffeine intake to get to this point. Nevertheless, scientists and health experts have developed some general guidelines for the safe use of caffeine, and there is always new information coming from research on caffeine.

In this book, we look at caffeine from the perspective of sports performance. We will find that although there is a history of caffeine use in sport, the science behind it is just decades old. Consequently, it is still on a reasonably steep learning curve that has been sidetracked at times. It is only recently that some new insights into caffeine and sports performance have allowed us to realize that it has more similarities to the general population's use of caffeine than we previously thought. There is a lot to learn from our knowledge and experiences of everyday caffeine use that could be applied to this specialized area.

Our journey through the caffeine story takes the following path. Chapter 1 presents a brief history lesson on the discovery of caffeine and the evolution of the drinks that provide the main sources of caffeine in our everyday eating patterns and social rituals. You'll also find some background information on how caffeine was used in sport and attracted the attention of exercise scientists over the decades preceding the 1980s, from where this book will pick up the tale in more detail.

Chapter 2 summarizes the way caffeine acts on our bodies at various levels of intake, trying to explain how it could enhance sports performance. This is a chapter with technical details that will not appeal to every reader. Feel free to skip it, but know that we have included this information because many athletes and coaches have developed a sophisticated interest in the chemistry and biochemistry behind supplements. At the very least, it may help you to make sense of the claims made by manufacturers of sport supplements, who often try to market their products by blinding with science (or quasi-science).

Chapter 3 will hopefully bring all readers back to the fold, providing information on where caffeine is found in both the general food supply and in specialized products and how much you can count on consuming from these sources. Explanations of the regulation of caffeine in foods and supplements around the world will help to explain why certain products are found in some countries but not others. In chapter 4, you'll learn how we've come to make use of these caffeine sources, by habit, accident, or design. We will summarize typical patterns of caffeine use in everyday diets as well as specific intakes by various populations, including athletes.

The next chapters of the book work through the questions that every athlete should ask when considering the use of a supplement: Does it work? Is it safe? Am I allowed to use it? In chapter 5, we delve into the modern research literature to isolate the studies on caffeine and exercise that have relevance to the real world of sports performance. We examine the evidence that caffeine enhances the performance of various types of sporting events, and we find which protocols of caffeine use (sources, doses, and timing of intake) provide consistent results. We'll even try to leave you with the tools to extract the bottom line from future studies of caffeine and sports performance.

Once you know whether caffeine is likely to offer benefits for your type of sport, you'll want to consider the information in chapter 6 on health risks, side effects, and general cautions associated with such caffeine use. Chapter 7 follows up with the position of caffeine in antidoping programs and the historical changes to this position. Caffeine in sport remains an area that is emotive and often misunderstood.

If, after reading the previous chapters, you have decided that you want to use caffeine to assist in the achievement of your training and competition goals, the final section of the book will help you to develop a personalized plan. Chapter 8 considers the effect that caffeine might have on other important elements of your preparation and recovery from exercise sessions—for example, hydration, sleep, and refueling. After all, your caffeine use needs to fit into the big picture of your goals. In chapter 9, you'll learn that your plan needs to account for potential factors that might alter the wanted and unwanted effects of caffeine. Some of these are fixed (e.g., sex, genetically determined response to caffeine), while others can be changed (e.g., background caffeine use, withdrawing from caffeine use for a couple of days, using it repeatedly, using it with other supplements).

Having all of this new knowledge is helpful, but it can be tricky to organize it into new practices. Therefore, chapter 10 provides the goods to help you put your personalized program together, using checklists to work through the issues for training and competition scenarios and offering tools to assemble and monitor the outcomes. We also describe a framework that might help the world of sport to develop a sensible and unified view of caffeine use by athletes.

Along the way, we will drop in quotes and anecdotes about the use and abuse of caffeine in sport. Some of this information is in the public domain, so we can name names. On other occasions, we provide some candid and personal insights about caffeine use from athletes we know, some of whom would rather not be identified due to the funny emotions that caffeine use seems to elicit in the general population. Finally, we will provide you with a reading list of the references we have consulted to write this book.

In summary, this book will provide you with the definitive *how*, *what*, and *why* or *why not* guide to the role of caffeine in your sport. We hope you enjoy our insights.

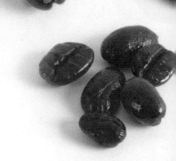

# Chapter

# 1

# A Brief History of Caffeine in Sport

Nearly 200 years ago, Friedlieb Ferdinand Runge, a 25-year-old German analytical chemist, isolated a special chemical in coffee beans. Shortly afterward, some French scientists working independently on a similar project produced the same results. Their work was inspired by scientific curiosity into the popularity of coffee drinking in Europe, a habit ingrained for several centuries; in fact, it often took place in special coffeehouses that could be seen as the Starbucks of their time. The unmistakable flavor and aroma of coffee were an obvious attraction, but it seemed that something more was involved. The effects seemed both euphoric and addictive. The newly identified compound was translated from German and French terms meaning "something from coffee" into the English word *caffeine*.

The discovery of caffeine suddenly began to make sense of many observations of human behavior dating back to the Stone Age. Across countries, cultures, and eras, there are consistent stories of people consuming parts of plants to provide an energy boost. Legends involve animals or people accidentally consuming a plant and subsequently experiencing wakefulness, elation, and vitality. With this discovery, consumption of the plant would become a ritual in the community. Tea leaves, cocoa beans, kola nuts, yerba maté, and guarana are all examples of this model. We now know that the common denominator of these and more than 60 other plant species is the presence of caffeine. And as far back as records exist, it seems that people have sought this natural stimulant to include in cultural and social activities, to enhance their performance of various pursuits, and to treat headaches, lethargy, and pain.

# History of Caffeine Use

Around the world, coffee and tea have become the major sources of caffeine intake. The preparation of coffee from roasted coffee beans apparently started in the Middle East in the 1400s before spreading to Europe around 1600 and then the Americas in the 1700s. The brewing of tea from tea leaves can be traced back to various Chinese dynasties from several centuries BC. However, globalization required the efforts of Marco Polo (1200s) and the Dutch East India Company (1600s), with tea drinking gaining popularity in Europe in the late 1600s and coffeehouses becoming fashionable from the 1600s onward. Although these establishments were primarily centers of social interaction, coffee and particularly tea were noted as tonics and used to treat a variety of ailments.

The evolution of the world's third most popular caffeine source, cola drinks, is an interesting tale involving both health and sport. Mineral waters from natural springs had been popular as both baths and beverages for centuries because of beliefs about their health-promoting properties. The late 1700s was the era of campaigns to produce a human-made version of these tonics. The first such glass of carbonated water was created by an English scientist, Dr. Joseph Priestley, who was also credited with the discovery of oxygen and carbon monoxide. Other scientists also found ways to achieve this feat, but their outcomes were always on a small scale.

It took the combination of a jeweler named Johann Jacob Schweppe, an engineer, and a scientist to perfect the process of making artificial mineral waters on a large scale, with Schweppe moving the successful business to England. Patents were established there and in the United States for "means to mass manufacture imitation mineral waters." One of these means was the soda fountain, and because mineral waters originated as a health tonic, the neighborhood pharmacy became the popular place to dispense sodas. Throughout the late 1800s, American pharmacists started to add medicinal or flavor-providing herbs to the unflavored drinks. This led to cola drinks, followed by the development of soda-producing companies with trademarked names and beverages, particularly Coca-Cola and Pepsi-Cola. Table 1.1 summarizes the origins of the two cola

**Table 1.1**  Origins of Cola Drinks*

| Beverage | Developed | Original ingredients | Original health claim |
|----------|-----------|----------------------|------------------------|
| Coca-Cola | 1886, Atlanta, Georgia | Sugar, lime, cinnamon, coca leaves, and kola nuts | Nerve and brain tonic, headache cure |
| Pepsi-Cola | 1898, New Bern, North Carolina | Vanilla, sugar, oils, pepsin, and kola nuts | Exhilarating and invigorating digestive aid, cure for dyspepsia |

*Information sourced from official drink manufacturer websites.

giants along with their original ingredients and health claims. When launched, Coca-Cola's two key ingredients were cocaine from the coca leaf and caffeine from the kola nut, explaining its name. Shortly after the turn of the century, it moved to using "spent" coca leaves from which the cocaine had been extracted, leaving caffeine as the only stimulant. The rest, as they say, is history.

The original marketing of cola beverages focused solely on their claimed medicinal properties. Soon, however, companies realized that people enjoyed consuming these drinks, and to increase sales, they wanted to remove the stigma associated with taking medicine. The focus of advertisements moved away from the concept of medicinal elixir and more toward life enhancer. Additionally, promotion and sponsorship became the tools to market expansion. This included aligning products with sport celebrities and other high-profile members of society.

In 1909, automobile racing pioneer Barney Oldfield became the first Pepsi celebrity endorser when he appeared in newspaper advertisements describing Pepsi-Cola as "A bully drink . . . refreshing, invigorating, a fine bracer for a race" (www.pepsiusa.com/faqs.php?section=highlights). In 1928, 1,000 cases of Coke traveled with the U.S. Olympic team to the Amsterdam Olympics. Coca-Cola has continued its association with the Olympic Games to this day: It is the longest continuous corporate partner, and it is a member of The Olympic Partner (TOP) program, the top-level sponsorship awarded to a handful of sponsors with exclusive worldwide marketing rights to the Winter and Summer Olympic Games. Around the world, PepsiCo and Coca-Cola continue to sponsor a large range of regional and international sporting events and teams, seeing sport sponsorship as a natural fit.

> Over the years I've fine-tuned a caffeine protocol that works for me. I take a small dose before the start and then use caffeinated gels in the second half of the race. Overall it adds up to around 250 mg of caffeine, which is less than many people get from their daily coffee habits. I take my prerace caffeine as a tablet, and I feel a bit funny about doing this in public. I know this isn't logical because it's probably less than the caffeine in a cup of coffee, but I feel that people judge it differently when it's in a pill.
>
> *Three-time Olympic medalist, distance event in track and field*

## History of Caffeine Use in Sport

It should come as no surprise that modern athletes and coaches were first attracted to caffeine because of its ability to clear the mind of fatigue and to act as a potential muscle stimulant. In the early days of modern sport (1900 onward), mixtures of plant-based stimulants were commonly used for performance enhancement.

Indeed, as discussed previously, many of these mixtures were available as tonics and patent medicines for use in the general population. Caffeine and cocaine were particularly popular additives because they were thought to stave off the fatigue and hunger brought on by prolonged exertion.

Throughout the early 1900s, caffeine was an ingredient in cocktails for athletes that included compounds such as cocaine, strychnine, ether, and heroin. Secret recipes developed by individual trainers, coaches, and athletes were designed to provide a competitive advantage over rivals. The use of pharmaceutical cocktails by endurance athletes was so common that one author described 6-day cycling races as "de facto experiments investigating the physiology of stress as well as the substances that might alleviate exhaustion" (Hoberman 2013). This situation continued until heroin and cocaine became prescription-only substances in the 1920s and, later, when sporting organizations developed antidoping programs in the 1960s.

The earliest published studies of the ergogenic (performance-enhancing) effects of caffeine also appeared at the start of the 20th century. William Rivers and Harald Webber, colleagues at the psychology laboratory at Cambridge University in the United Kingdom, undertook a series of experiments between 1903 and 1908 on the influence of caffeine on the capacity to perform muscular work. As was common at the time, they used themselves as subjects. Their investigations included many of the elements we now consider important in sport science research, such as the use of ergometers to measure some aspect of physical activity (in this case, an ergogram, which measured the ability to lift a weight repeatedly with a finger or hand) and standardization of diet and exercise (they avoided caffeine and alcohol for months, if not years, before their experiments). Remarkably, they described the phenomenon that part of the mental and physical effects achieved by taking a compound were caused by the psychological excitement of knowing that one was indulging. This led them to employ double-blind, placebo-controlled procedures where neither the subject nor the researcher was aware of whether the experiment involved caffeine or a placebo until the conclusion of the entire study. However, today's critical eye would note that they had small subject numbers and an artificial measurement of exercise performance.

It wasn't until the 1940s that significant research on caffeine and exercise performance started to appear. American researchers from the Northwestern University medical school investigated the effects of intravenous infusions of caffeine on the capacity to perform and recover from rapidly exhausting work. These studies were significant in that they used a cycle ergometer (a more applied exercise task), had larger groups of participants (one study had 23 subjects!), and considered variables of importance such as whether subjects were trained or untrained.

John Haldi and Winfrey Wynn, from Emory University in Atlanta, Georgia, studied the influence of caffeine (250 mg) on swimming performance (91 m or 100 yd). They failed to show any influence of caffeine on performance or fatigue. Danish researchers from the University of Copenhagen investigated the effects of a range of stimulants (300 mg caffeine, alcohol, cocaine, strychnine, and nitroglycerin) on cycling performance lasting from 15 s to 5 min. Of all the drugs tested, only caffeine improved performance slightly and only in the test with the longest duration.

In the late 1970s, a series of studies from the Human Performance Laboratory at Ball State University under the wing of the father of sport nutrition, Dave Costill, investigated the benefits of caffeine intake (250-300 mg) on cycling endurance and performance. This coincided with the running boom and precipitated new interest and popular use of caffeine in endurance sports. Continued research on caffeine and exercise has intensified in three major areas: the interactive effects of caffeine and exercise on body metabolism, the effect of caffeine on prolonged exercise and sleep deprivation with relevance to military operations, and the effect of caffeine on sports performance. This is the era of the science and practice of caffeine use in sport that is covered in this book.

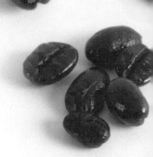

# Chapter
............
# 2

# How Caffeine Works

As we have seen in chapter 1, caffeine is a naturally occurring chemical found in certain plants. Furthermore, as we will explore in chapter 3, it has become an additive in a range of foods and drinks. Caffeine has no nutritive value, but its druglike qualities explain centuries of use by humans to prevent or alleviate pain and general fatigue. It is also a habit-forming compound that appears to cause both physical and psychological dependencies. Withdrawal from regular caffeine use causes headaches and other symptoms, but these are relatively minor in comparison with many other habit-forming drugs such as alcohol, nicotine, morphine, cocaine, and opium.

## Metabolism of Caffeine

It is difficult to discuss the actions of caffeine in the body without some kind of immersion in chemistry and physiology. Bear with us or simply skip this chapter. In chemical terms, caffeine is an alkaloid, which means it is a basic and organic plant-derived substance, with the chemical name of 1,3,7-trimethylxanthine. It is an odorless white powder that is soluble in both water and lipids and has a bitter taste.

The chemical structure of caffeine is similar to that of adenosine, a very biologically active compound in the body. Adenosine can act alone or bound to other chemicals, most noticeably as the backbone for adenosine triphosphate (ATP), the most important form of usable energy in the body. Among its range of functions, adenosine is involved in the dilation or opening up of blood vessels and the release of hormones and fuels from tissues. It also acts as a cell-signaling molecule. Caffeine can bind to the adenosine receptors that are found throughout the body, and in most cases, as we will discuss later, this binding antagonizes (works against) the actions of adenosine.

When caffeine is consumed, it appears in the blood rapidly, with peak values reported within 45 to 90 min. Blood concentrations of caffeine are related to the size of the dose that was consumed. With drugs and many other compounds, we usually rate the dose according to the size (body mass or BM) of the person who consumes it. In the case of caffeine, the ingestion of 3 milligrams per kilogram of body mass (hereafter simply noted as mg/kg) produces blood levels of ~15 to 20 micromoles per liter (μM), while ingesting 6mg/kg produces levels of ~40 to 50 μM, and consuming 9 mg/kg results in concentrations of ~60 to 75 μM.

Examples of blood caffeine profiles after consuming such doses are found in figure 2.1. Of course, in many studies like the one that produced the results in this figure, the blood caffeine concentrations were achieved by consuming caffeine in capsule form as a single dose. If, as in real life, caffeine is ingested in a drink such as coffee, tea, or cola, it is generally spread out over a period of time. Although this would cause a delayed entry of caffeine in the blood, peak blood caffeine levels are generally still reached in 45 to 90 min.

Although the caffeine dose has been described according to the size of the person, a secondary reference point is the absolute amount that can be found in foods and drinks. Assuming the subject weighed 70 kg, the doses seen in the study would equate to about 210, 420, and 630 mg of caffeine for the 3, 6, and 9 mg/kg doses. Chapter 3 will show that the larger two doses constitute a lot of caffeine in terms of common dietary sources.

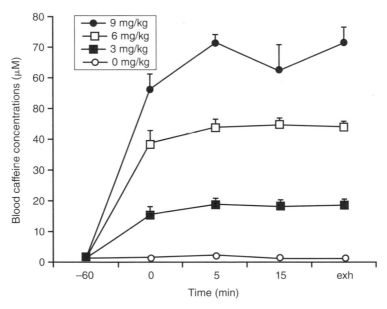

**Figure 2.1**   Blood caffeine concentrations following the intake of caffeine doses equal to 0, 3, 6 and 9 mg/kg.

Reprinted from T.E. Graham and L.L. Spriet, "Metabolic, catecholamine, and exercise performance responses to various doses of caffeine," *Journal of Applied Psychology* 78(3): 867-874.

Once it is ingested, caffeine is slowly metabolized or degraded in the liver with a half-life of 3.5 to 5 hours. This means that only half of the original caffeine in the blood remains after 3.5 to 5 hours, and then in the next 3.5 to 5 hours, another half of the caffeine is gone, leaving about 25% of the original amount, and so forth. So, there still can be traces of caffeine in the blood 24 hours after ingestion. There is also a large variation in the rate at which individuals break down caffeine. Not all caffeine is broken down, however. About 0.5% to 3% of the dose is excreted, unchanged, in the urine. This is the basis of urine tests for caffeine intake (see Urinary Caffeine Concentrations: A Poor Way to Measure Caffeine Intake).

The breakdown of caffeine begins with the removal of the methyl groups by a family of liver enzymes called the *cytochrome P-450 oxygenases*. Some drugs or chemicals found naturally in food affect the activity of these liver enzymes, meaning that they can slow down or speed up the process of caffeine breakdown. There is also some genetic variability in the activity of this liver pathway. This is just one of the reasons why different people experience different outcomes from the same dose of caffeine or the same person can have a different reaction to a caffeine dose—depending on the breakdown pattern of caffeine, it may hang around in the bloodstream in high concentrations for a long time or it may be cleared quickly.

The by-products of the breakdown of caffeine appear within minutes of consumption and include paraxanthine (85%), theobromine (10%), and theophylline (5%). Why should you care about these chemicals? For one thing, they have the ability to exert their own physiological effects on the body. In addition, they are found in smaller amounts in some common caffeine-containing beverages; for instance, tea contains a reasonable amount of theophylline and chocolate contains some theobromine. If you read labels on supplements, you might also find them as ingredients in some multicomponent products sold for weight loss or as preworkout stimulants.

## General Effects on the Body

The quick release of caffeine into the bloodstream, followed by its slow metabolism, means that a dose of caffeine has plenty of time to exert its effects on the body. Importantly, it can cross the blood–brain barrier, the resistant barrier that blood vessels in the wall of the brain impose to stop compounds from moving into the cerebral spinal fluid. Therefore, caffeine should be able to interact with every tissue in the body, either by interacting with receptors on the surface of the tissue or actually gaining entry into the cell in question.

As described earlier, the most common way caffeine exerts its effects is through its ability to compete for the adenosine receptors found in many parts

# Urinary Caffeine Concentrations:
# A Poor Way to Measure Caffeine Intake

Both in real life and in laboratory studies, there has been a need to be able to characterize a person's recent caffeine intake. Taking blood samples always adds a level of complexity or logistical difficulty to any activity, so urine measures have become the default method. What's being measured is the caffeine that has not been metabolized within the body but has instead been excreted, unchanged, into the urine. According to pharmacokinetic studies, this accounts for about 0.5% to 3% of any caffeine dose. In the case of urine tests for caffeine use in a sporting competition, an athlete simply needs to urinate into a special jar at some time after the event. The sample goes to a lab and the caffeine concentration is measured. What could go wrong?

In fact, plenty. Both logic and experience have uncovered major flaws in the idea that such a urine test can pinpoint an individual's specific caffeine use. To begin with, there is the variability between people in the amount of caffeine that escapes metabolism. Although the difference between excretion rates might seem small, the relative differences are high. For example, if two people consume the same caffeine dose, the one who excretes 3% of the dose will produce six times as much caffeine in their urine as the person with the 0.5% loss. And that's just the start, because this caffeine is found as a concentration in urine, which has its own variability in production. Professor Don Birkett from Flinders University in Adelaide undertook a study that tracked urinary caffeine concentrations in young volunteers following a steady intake of caffeine over 6 days. Urinary caffeine concentrations varied 16-fold among subjects, sometimes exceeding 12 µg/ml, which at the time of the study was the threshold above which an athlete would be deemed to have used caffeine as a prohibited substance (see chapter 7).

Finally, there is the problem of the lack of standardization in the collection of urine samples in antidoping programs. Recent caffeine use might be better tracked if, for example, a 24-hour urine collection was undertaken to pool all the caffeine in all the urine. However, doping control is based on the collection of a spot urine sample at the athlete's convenience in the hours after an event. Depending on the type of sport, it could be just after a race lasting a minute or in the recovery from a competition lasting 8 hours. Furthermore, the athlete may have taken their caffeine dose an hour before the race or throughout the event. He or she may have urinated several times during the race (and even afterward) or not at all since getting up that morning. Are you still feeling confident that we are measuring the same thing each time?

This process might be a reasonable and pragmatic method to test for the absence or presence of substances in urine where even tiny amounts denote the absolute intake of a prohibited substance. However, the frailty of the process to be able to quantify the intake of a specific amount of caffeine is now recognized. This was one reason why caffeine was removed from the list of prohibited substances (chapter 7).

of the body. When a molecule of the caffeine binds to an adenosine receptor, it stops adenosine from binding, thereby preventing adenosine from exerting its normal effect. This is referred to as *adenosine antagonism*. By counteracting the many functions that adenosine exerts in many tissues, caffeine has profound and varied effects on our bodies. We will now examine a few of these adenosine-mediated effects.

> The England right-back Glen Johnson told BBC 5 Live after Wednesday's 1-1 draw with Poland that some of the players had taken caffeine pills before the postponed World Cup qualifier and then had trouble sleeping. "I'm not blaming that at all but it's obviously not done you any favours. . . . A lot of the lads take ProPlus [caffeine] tablets before the game and we all took that for the game [on Tuesday] then the game is off and no one can sleep."
>
> *Sam Wallace (2012)*

## Effects on the Adrenal Medulla

The adrenal medulla is the core of the adrenal gland, an important organ found near the kidney. It releases several hormones into the bloodstream that belong to a family often called *stress hormones* or *catecholamines*. The adrenal medulla is responsible for producing 80% of the body's epinephrine (also called *adrenaline*) and 20% of the norepinephrine (also called *noradrenaline*). These hormones are responsible for mobilizing the body into action in response to stress, also known as the fight-or-flight phenomenon. This includes mobilizing fuels to provide the muscles with energy, increasing the heart rate and the force of heart muscle contractions, constricting blood vessels in areas that are nonessential during exercise (such as the gut and noncontracting muscle), and increasing alertness. At lower caffeine doses (1.5-3 mg/kg), there is generally no effect on epinephrine levels in the blood, and even at moderate to high doses (5-9 mg/kg), there is little effect on norepinephrine levels. Meanwhile at the high end of this range, caffeine increases epinephrine concentrations at rest and exercise by about 50% to 100%, possibly because caffeine interferes with processes that would normally limit epinephrine release.

## Effects on Adipose Tissue

The body uses energy from a mixture of fuel sources, particularly from its fat and carbohydrate stores. How much each fuel source contributes to the mix is determined by complex factors, including how much is available and how quickly it needs to be used. Obviously, exercise is one of the conditions in which the rate of fuel use increases (often dramatically) and in which some stores can run out, especially muscle carbohydrate stores. Caffeine is one of the factors that can alter fuel use in some people. We used to think this was an important finding to explain the benefits of caffeine on sports performance. As we shall see, however, it isn't a universal finding in all people, and caffeine enhances performance in exercise situations that aren't limited by fuel use. All in all, this finding is of interest, but it might not be as critical as we once thought.

Most of us have relatively large amounts of body fat stored in our adipose tissue, but its availability for fuel use is regulated in part by the rate at which the fat is broken down to release free fatty acids into the bloodstream for delivery to the muscles. When we are sedentary, the rate of free fatty acid release from adipose tissue is low and is arranged by the combined effects of low catecholamine levels and the presence of adenosine and insulin. Both adenosine and insulin bind to receptors on the surface of adipose tissue and inhibit the processes that break down and release fat into the blood. When fuel needs increase, for example during exercise, the rate of fat release can be greatly elevated via increases in blood epinephrine and norepinephrine levels.

In some people, caffeine can cancel out adenosine's ability to keep fatty acid levels low in the bloodstream. Sometimes caffeine actually achieves this by directly affecting the adipose tissue, independent of the work of adenosine. One way or another, in some people, caffeine leads to an increased breakdown of adipose tissue and an accumulation of fatty acids in the blood. But caffeine does not increase resting levels of fatty acids in everyone; in fact, the results vary quite a lot from person to person, and the effect is even less frequent when the caffeine dose is less than 3 mg/kg. Generally, when such variation is seen in any physiological system, we talk about dividing people into responders (those who see a large effect) and nonresponders (those who have a nonexistent or trivial outcome). When this response is examined in a study that involves a mixture of responders and nonresponders, the results of the group tend to cancel each other out so that no clear outcomes are seen. This explains the apparent contradictions among the results of various studies.

Increased blood levels of fatty acids generally lead to increased use of fat as a muscle fuel. This claimed fat-burning effect of caffeine was promoted in several ways. The first alleged benefit was as an agent for weight loss—an effect that hasn't held up to scrutiny for a variety of reasons. The second alleged benefit, heavily promoted in sport nutrition until recently, was the positioning of fat as an alternative fuel source to spare the use of the limited stores of carbohydrate fuel (glycogen) in the muscles. During the 1970s, scientists became aware of the importance of muscle glycogen as a fuel for prolonged or high-intensity exercise. It was well known that depletion of muscle glycogen was associated with fatigue and a decline in exercise performance, so efforts were made to safeguard the muscle against this occurrence. Strategies to increase muscle glycogen stores (carbohydrate loading) were shown to be effective in enhancing performance by delaying the point of fuel depletion. A second approach was to reduce the rate of glycogen utilization. If caffeine could increase fat utilization during exercise, it would allow glycogen stores to be used at a slower rate and be available at the end of longer exercise tasks and sporting events. This became the standard theory to explain observations of better performance in marathons and other lengthy exercise activities following caffeine intake.

By the mid-1990s, however, evidence began to accumulate that glycogen sparing wasn't a major mechanism behind the ergogenic effects of caffeine. First, as we have explained, scientists realized that the fat-mobilizing and glycogen-sparing effects of caffeine are not universal. Second, it was discovered that even in people who do respond to caffeine by releasing more fat into the blood, this effect is gone after 10 to 15 minutes of exercise. Thus it would not seem to be sufficient to explain the improved performance in a long event or exercise task. Finally, an examination of individual participants in studies found that performance benefits were seen in both the responders and nonresponders to caffeine-stimulated fat release, and that caffeine is of benefit to short-duration exercise that isn't limited by the size of muscle glycogen stores.

The bottom line is that the reliable observations of work-enhancing effects during prolonged aerobic exercise could no longer be attributed to greater fat use and muscle glycogen sparing. It was time to accept that the effects of caffeine on the central nervous system (CNS) appeared to provide a more plausible theory for the ergogenic effects of caffeine, especially when consumed at low doses.

> An elite runner, a non-coffee drinker, once told me when he first heard about caffeine being an ergogenic aid, he drank two cups prerace on an empty stomach. Along the lines of if some is good, then more is better. That ruined that race!
>
> *Sports dietitian and author of sports nutrition books*

## Effects on the Brain

It is widely accepted that caffeine is a CNS stimulant, causing increased wakefulness, arousal, vigilance, and alertness as well as improved mood. Because caffeine can freely pass through the blood–brain barrier, its consumption causes a rapid rise in caffeine concentration in the brain and CNS in concert with changes in other body tissues. Studies on rats show that caffeine increases the concentration of brain neurotransmitters—the chemicals released from a brain cell (neuron) to talk to neighboring neurons—increasing the firing rate of neurons in the brain and increasing spontaneous movement. The brain has high numbers of adenosine receptors, so it is generally accepted that caffeine causes the increase in neurotransmitters via the adenosine antagonism effect.

In the brain, adenosine acts as both a neurotransmitter and a chemical that affects the release of other neurotransmitters (i.e., it is a neuromodulator). Generally, the presence of adenosine and adenosine-like compounds reduces motor activity, decreases wakefulness and vigilance, and decreases the concentrations of other stimulatory neurotransmitters. Caffeine and other adenosine receptor antagonists have the opposite effect by blocking the adenosine receptors.

There are some curious issues, however. Caffeine has been shown to increase the concentration, synthesis, and turnover of all major neurotransmitters, including serotonin, dopamine, acetylcholine, norepinephrine, and glutamate. The consequences of increasing the levels of these neurotransmitters are currently unknown. However, some neurotransmitters, such as dopamine and serotonin, have been implicated in *causing* fatigue in the CNS, so it is not clear how, if caffeine increases all neurotransmitter concentrations, it could *alleviate* fatigue. One suggestion is that the caffeine-induced increases in excitatory neurotransmitters might dominate those causing fatigue, with the balance sheet leading to increased alertness and arousal, alleviating fatigue. Another possible explanation involves the existence of several types (called *isoforms*) of adenosine receptors. Each type might have different affinities for adenosine and caffeine and respond differently in terms of releasing neurotransmitters.

It is difficult to investigate what is occurring inside the brain. However, some recent work on animals has supported the argument that the work-enhancing effects of caffeine occur mainly via its actions on the CNS. A study from the University of South Carolina involved rats that had been trained to run on a treadmill and had a catheter implanted into their brain by which they could receive direct injections of chemicals into the brain. Each rat undertook four trials, each receiving a different treatment 30 min before they ran to fatigue on a treadmill. The treatments were caffeine, which was expected to block the effects of adenosine; a chemical called *NECA*, which acts like adenosine; caffeine and NECA together; and a control trial of injection fluid only.

Figure 2.2 shows the effects of the various treatments on running endurance. Compared with the control treatment, caffeine injections improved run time by about 60%, while NECA impaired run time by 68%. When caffeine and NECA were given together, they essentially cancelled each other out, producing a run time that was the same as the control trial. A particularly important finding was that measurements of activities outside the brain (muscle glycogen use and blood concentrations of fatty acids, glucose, and stress hormones) did not differ among the four trials. In addition, when the same experiment was repeated, only this time with the injection of the same four chemicals into the body cavity, there was no difference in the run times to exhaustion. Together, these results demonstrate that the important effects of caffeine occur in the brain and that performance can be improved without any metabolic effects on the muscle.

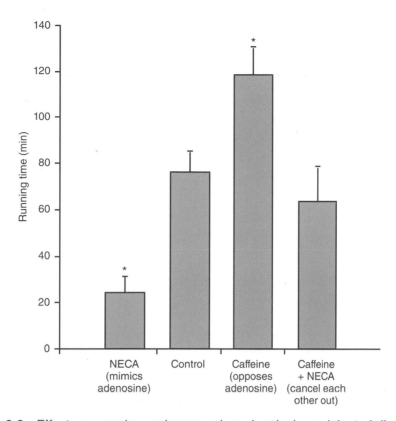

**Figure 2.2**   Effects on running endurance when chemicals are injected directly into the brains of rats.

Reprinted, by permission, from J.M. Davis, Z. Zhao, H.S. Stock, et al., 2003, "Central nervous system effects of caffeine and adenosine on fatigue," *American Journal of Physiology - Regulatory, Integrative and Comparative Physiology* 284: R399-R404.

Other human studies have provided intriguing results that relate to the brain and caffeine. In 2002 we published a study from work done at the Australian Institute of Sport (AIS) to investigate why elite athletes consume flat cola drinks in the last part of long sporting events such as marathons and road cycling races (see chapter 5 for more details). To be honest, we thought these athletes were crazy because the doses of caffeine were very low and the timing was all wrong compared with the scientist's traditional approach to the ergogenic use of caffeine (6 mg/kg dose taken 1 hour before the event). In fact, the athletes proved us wrong—the cola improved time-trial performance by 3%, the same magnitude of performance enhancement seen with the traditional caffeine protocol. We were able to determine that the effects of the cola drink were partially explained by extra carbohydrate intake but mostly by the caffeine dose. Surprisingly, the total caffeine intake provided by the cola drink was only 133 mg or ~1.9 mg/kg, resulting in plasma caffeine levels of less than 10 μM. We couldn't find any evidence of physiological responses to caffeine in adipose tissue or the muscle.

This suggests that the beneficial effects of caffeine were being directed to the CNS late in exhaustive exercise.

A follow-up study at the University of Guelph looked at the effects of two low doses of caffeine using a similar exercise and caffeine protocol—caffeine consumed in the last third of a steady-state ride before undertaking a time trial. The caffeine doses were 100 or 200 mg, equal to ~1.5 and 3.0 mg/kg. Again, even with these low intakes, subjects completed the time trial significantly faster (by nearly 3% for the 1.5 mg/kg dose and another 4% for the 3.0 mg/kg dose). Plasma caffeine levels reached only 14 μM in the 100 mg dose trial and 25 μM in the 200 mg dose trial. Again, there were no differences in the physiological responses to exercise in terms of heart rate, fuel use, blood concentrations of substrates, and stress hormones after the caffeine doses, further supporting the hypothesis that low levels of caffeine late in prolonged exercise work through the CNS to improve exercise performance.

These findings also provide a strong argument that the brain may be more sensitive to caffeine when it is already fatigued. In these circumstances, even a little caffeine can have a large effect. Of course, many of us have observed this finding in our everyday use of caffeine. When we are brain-dead from writing reports or sitting in a lecture or meeting, we know that a single serving of a caffeinated beverage can quickly perk us up for a second effort. It's strange that even though we had noticed that a small amount of caffeine allowed us to gather ourselves together after a hard day at the office and galvanize our efforts for postwork activities, we hadn't thought to apply this knowledge to the more specialized area of sports performance until quite recently. As we will see in chapter 5, the new thinking with caffeine and sport is that small doses can produce quick and powerful effects in many people, especially when it is consumed when fatigue is starting to set in.

In the absence of being able to directly measure what is happening inside the human brain during exercise, sport scientists rely on having subjects rate how hard it feels to complete the sport or exercise task using the rating of perceived exertion (RPE). This scale goes from 1 to 20, where low numbers coincide with feelings of light exertion and the highest number coincides with maximal exertion. It can be applied to the whole-body feeling or to specific areas—for example, to the feeling of breathing or the feeling in one's legs. Several studies have demonstrated that RPE is lower when subjects are asked to run or cycle at a given power output following caffeine ingestion compared with a placebo or control condition. Alternatively, when subjects are asked to work at the same RPE during an exercise activity, studies often find that caffeine intake produces higher outputs or exercise intensity.

It has been speculated that the ability of caffeine to reduce the perception of how hard we are working is due to a decrease in the firing threshold of motor neurons or changes in muscle contraction force. Both mechanisms would reduce

## Stop the Presses

### Caffeine: Brain Messages Straight From the Mouth?

Just as this book was going to press, a new publication from a consortium involving the UK Sports Council grabbed our attention. It reported on studies in which caffeine had been provided to athletes in the form of a mouth rinse. This adds to the vast literature showing that simply swilling a carbohydrate drink around your mouth can enhance pacing and performance in shorter endurance events (~60 min duration). The explanation is cool—receptors in the mouth that sense that carbohydrate is on the way then directly communicate to specific parts of the brain that make you feel good and better able to exercise at sustained high intensity. The carbohydrate doesn't even have to be consumed to impart the benefit—in fact, swilling it around for 5 seconds appears to be more effective than quickly swallowing it. The new paper from Martyn Beaven and colleagues suggests that a similar effect appears to occur with caffeine. Their study involved recreationally trained athletes who undertook a protocol of 6 high-intensity cycling sprints interspersed with 24 seconds of recovery. Caffeinated mouth rinse, which was swilled just before each of the sprints before being spat out, appeared to improve power outputs in the first sprint in the series both alone and when combined with carbohydrate. More work is needed to repeat these findings and to ensure that the caffeine is simply hitting receptors in the mouth that talk to the brain rather than being absorbed into the blood according to our traditional understanding of caffeine. But it confirms the finding that the brain is truly a remarkable organ in the way it responds to a variety of stimuli.

the feedback sent by the muscle to the brain—that is, the muscle would tell the brain that the contractions were easier to achieve. However, in many cases the blood caffeine levels associated with the reduced feeling of effort do not appear to be high enough to cause these types of changes at the level of the muscle and the nerves that act on it. Over the course of a prolonged exercise task, there is a decline in the neural ability to generate maximal voluntary force and an increase in the central drive needed to maintain a given intensity of exercise. In other words, the muscle can't keep producing the same force or power and the brain has to work harder to keep the muscles producing the same outcomes. Caffeine has been shown to improve central drive by increasing spinal excitability, self-sustained firing, and voluntary activation, all leading to increased maximal force. Thus, although the caffeine concentrations in the blood may be too low to directly affect the ability of the muscles to contract, they may be high enough to maintain or improve the ability of the brain to activate the muscles.

Another explanation of the lower RPE findings following caffeine intake might be that the same amount of feedback sent from the contracting muscles is interpreted in the brain as less forceful or as less painful. In support of this is a significant body of literature that has examined the pain-reducing capacity of caffeine during various forms of exercise. Most of these studies have reported reductions in leg pain at a given power output following moderate doses (5-6 mg/kg) of caffeine given 1 hour before exercise. However, two reports used lower doses (2-3 mg/kg) of caffeine consumed before exercise and failed to find any pain-reducing effects in neutral and cool environments. There do not appear to be any studies that have examined the pain-numbing effects of consuming low caffeine doses during exercise.

A final hypothesis for the decreased perception of effort is that caffeine may directly affect the release of beta-endorphins and other hormones that modulate the feelings of discomfort and pain associated with intense and exhaustive exercise. Surprisingly, little work has been done in this area.

## Effects on the Muscle

Caffeine appears to have other effects on exercise that do not derive from activities related to adenosine receptors. Some of these effects include direct actions on the muscle. It helps to have a good understanding of the biochemistry involved in muscle contractions to appreciate these effects. It is hard to avoid technical terms in explaining this, so this section may only appeal to those with some knowledge of exercise physiology. It should also be noted that the evidence for these ideas comes from test-tube experiments on pieces of muscle that are bathed in high concentrations of caffeine. Therefore, there may be some problems in translating the findings to intact human beings and real-life sport.

The most likely pathway by which caffeine might directly benefit muscle contractions is via an increased release of calcium ($Ca^{2+}$) inside the muscle cell, which triggers it to contract and produce force. One cause of fatigue during exercise is the gradual reduction in the amount of calcium released each time we want the muscles to contract. If caffeine could increase the release of calcium, we might be able to fight off fatigue for a little longer. A second mechanism for caffeine involves the muscle membrane potential, which relates to the amounts of sodium ($Na^+$) and potassium ($K^+$) on each side of the muscle membrane. An enzyme ($Na^+$-$K^+$ ATPase) is responsible for pumping $Na^+$ and $K^+$ back and forth across the membrane to achieve the membrane potential needed for muscle contraction. Once again, when this enzyme seems to lose some of its activity during exercise, the membrane potential is not correct and the muscle doesn't contract as well. By preserving the activity of the enzyme and membrane potential, caffeine may have a second direct effect on reducing muscle fatigue.

These effects have been seen when experiments are done with the equivalent of muscle in a test tube. However, the concentrations of caffeine needed to produce these effects are still well above the highest blood caffeine levels seen in humans following a dose of caffeine. So, despite the theoretical promise, it seems unlikely that these direct effects of caffeine on activating muscle contractions are a major player in sports performance. This is especially the case considering that, as shown throughout the book, low levels of caffeine are ergogenic.

There have also been some experiments suggesting that caffeine may improve the availability of carbohydrate fuel for the muscle. This may arise from enhancement of the process of moving or transporting glucose into the muscle cells or from activating the enzyme that breaks down glycogen stores into glucose. However, these actions may only be important in test-tube experiments, because real-life exercise provides a number of signals that activate these processes when appropriate without needing to rely on caffeine.

Finally, there has been much scientific discussion about the ability of caffeine to inhibit an enzyme called *phosphodiesterase*. This enzyme normally breaks down a chemical called *cyclic AMP*, which is an important signaling molecule in many cells. It is produced when either epinephrine or norepinephrine binds to its receptors in any cell of the body. We have previously explained that these hormones are responsible for mobilizing the body for the fight-or-flight phenomenon. However, the concentrations needed to show these effects in test-tube studies are much higher than anything athletes would ever experience in their blood after caffeine ingestion. So, this theory of action by caffeine on the body seems theoretical rather than practical.

## Effects on Glucose Absorption

Some evidence suggests that caffeine can increase the gut absorption of glucose. This could mean that when carbohydrate is consumed during exercise, a greater amount gets delivered to the muscle to provide an additional fuel source. Several studies have looked at the practical aspects of this. One study from the Netherlands had well-trained subjects cycle for 90 minutes at ~70% $\dot{V}O_2$max after an overnight fast on three occasions. Just before exercise and at 20 and 40 min into exercise, the subjects ingested either water, a sport drink (~7% carbohydrate), or the sport drink and ~100 mg caffeine. They reported that the caffeine condition increased intestinal glucose absorption by 23% over the other two conditions.

Another study had overnight-fasted and well-trained subjects exercise for 2 hours at ~55% $\dot{V}O_2$max on three occasions: water ingestion only (~1.65 L), ingestion of the same volume of a carbohydrate solution (~48 g/h), or the carbohydrate solution with caffeine (10 mg/kg over 2 h). Oxidation of the carbohydrate consumed during the final 30 minutes of

Cyclist Steve Hegg was disqualified from competing at the 1988 Olympic Games in Seoul because of a positive drug test for caffeine. Hegg was due to be a member of the Olympic track cycling pursuit team, having earned a silver medal in this event and a gold medal in the individual pursuit at the 1984 Los Angeles Olympic Games.

exercise was 26% higher in the caffeine trial. The authors attributed this result to increased intestinal absorption, although the benefit could have occurred at other steps in the pathway between carbohydrate intake and muscle fuel use (e.g., stomach emptying, uptake of glucose into the liver, muscle glucose uptake).

Because this investigation used high levels of caffeine and did not measure performance, the study was repeated under conditions that were more applicable to sport, using an exercise protocol that simulated an event to a greater extent and used a lower caffeine dose. Well-trained subjects cycled for 105 minutes at ~62% $\dot{V}O_2$max and then performed a time trial that required the completion of a fixed amount of work as quickly as possible (~45 minutes) on three occasions: drinking a placebo solution, ingesting a carbohydrate solution (43 g/h), or ingesting the carbohydrate solution with 5.3 mg/kg caffeine. The lower caffeine dose enhanced performance but did not change the oxidation of carbohydrate from the drink consumed during exercise. In a final study, cyclists ingested a placebo or 1.5 or 3 mg/kg 1 hour before exercise. They then rode for 120 minutes at ~70% $\dot{V}O_2$max followed by a time trial. There were no differences in the contribution of a carbohydrate drink (consumed during the cycling protocol) to muscle fuel use between trials.

Collectively, these results argue that a high dose of caffeine is required to increase carbohydrate absorption and oxidation during prolonged exercise, and these findings are not present when moderate to low doses of caffeine are consumed. This again suggests that the performance-enhancing effects of low doses of caffeine are not due to metabolic effects but rather direct effects on the brain.

## The Bottom Line

Caffeine can have many effects on the body, but the most powerful and widespread appear to occur as a result of caffeine blocking the actions of a chemical called *adenosine*. It is difficult to know which of these effects contributes the most to the work-enhancing and fatigue-alleviating effects of caffeine, but the strongest evidence suggests that the CNS is the main target. This is especially true given the recent evidence that small doses of caffeine can be very ergogenic, especially late in prolonged and fatiguing exercise. It also seems that many sites in the CNS are positively affected by caffeine. The outcomes include the maintenance of our will to keep exercising (central drive), the sustained ability of the muscle to contract and produce force, and the reduced perception of messages of pain or fatigue sent by the muscles back to the brain.

Who would have thought that a compound that is so readily available could produce so many powerful outcomes and so much mystery about how it does it? The time is now right to learn where caffeine can be found in our diets and how much we are likely to consume by accident or design.

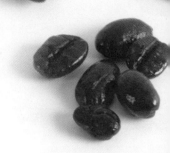

Chapter
• • • • • • • • • • • •

# 3

# Finding Caffeine in Our Diets

E ach day, most adults consume some caffeine. This is usually voluntary—in fact, it's often consumed with a sense of urgency. Nevertheless, because it is so engrained in our lives and food supply, some people may consume caffeine without realizing it.

Around the world, caffeine is most commonly consumed as a natural ingredient found in coffee, tea, cola beverages, and chocolate. However, the list of other sources of caffeine or guarana (a South American plant containing high levels of caffeine) is long and growing. It includes

- nonprescription medications;
- energy drinks, energy-drink concentrates (shots), and energy ice blocks;
- premixed alcoholic drinks;
- confectionery such as sweets and gums;
- sport foods such as drinks, waters, bars, and gels;
- dietary supplements; and even
- nasal sprays!

The arrival of these newer sources of caffeine has been a cause of concern for some people but a world of new possibilities for others. Either way, it has increased the ways in which caffeine can form part of our everyday diets or be taken specifically to achieve better performance in sport.

Table 3.1 summarizes the caffeine content of common foods and drinks in typical serving sizes, while table 3.2 summarizes the caffeine content of sport foods, supplements, and other nonprescription pharmaceutical products. We have identified which of these values represent the independent analysis of the

**Table 3.1** Caffeine Content of Common Foods, Drinks, and Therapeutic Products From a Variety of Sources†

| Food or drink | Serving size | Caffeine content (mg) |
| --- | --- | --- |
| COFFEE AND TEA PRODUCTS | | |
| Instant coffee | 250 ml cup | 60 (12-169)* |
| Brewed coffee | 250 ml cup | 80 (40-110)* |
| Brewed coffee (same outlet on different days) | 250 ml cup | 130-282* |
| Short black coffee/espresso from variety of outlets (AUS) | 1 standard serving | 107 (25-214)* |
| Starbucks Breakfast Blend brewed coffee (USA) | 600 ml (venti size) | 415 (256-564)* |
| Iced coffee—commercial brands (AUS) | 500 ml bottle | 30-200, depending on brand |
| Starbucks Double Shot coffee drink | 192 ml can | 130 |
| Starbucks Double Shot (energy varieties) | 240 ml can | 78 |
| Frappuccino | 375 ml cup | 90 |
| Tea | 250 ml cup | 27 (9-51)* |
| Black tea | 250 ml cup | 25-110 |
| Green tea | 250 ml cup | 30-50 |
| Iced tea | 600 ml bottle | 20-40 |
| CHOCOLATE | | |
| Hot chocolate | 250 ml cup | 5-10 |
| Chocolate—milk | 60 g | 5-15 |
| Chocolate—dark | 60 g | 10-50 |
| Viking chocolate bar | 60 g | 58 |
| SOFT DRINKS/SODA BEVERAGES | | |
| Coca-Cola and Coke Zero | 355 ml can | 34 |
| Diet Coke | 355 ml can | 46 |
| Pepsi | 355 ml can | 38 |
| Pepsi Max | 355 ml can | 68 |
| Mountain Dew (all varieties other than decaf or Game Fuel) | 355 ml can | 36 |
| Mountain Dew (Game Fuel varieties) | 355 ml can | 48 |
| Dr. Pepper | 355 ml can | 40 |
| RC Cola | 355 ml can | 36 |
| Canada Dry Cola (not diet) | 355 ml can | 30 |
| ENERGY DRINKS | | |
| Red Bull energy drink | 250 ml can | 80 |
| V energy drink (AUS/NZ) | 500 ml can | 155 |
| Mother energy drink (Aus/NZ)/Relentless energy drink (UK) | 500 ml can | 160 |
| Monster energy drink | 500 ml can | 160 |
| Lipovitan energy drink | 250 ml can | 50 |
| Rockstar energy drink | 500 ml can | 160 |

| Food or drink | Serving size | Caffeine content (mg) |
|---|---|---|
| ENERGY DRINKS *(continued)* | | |
| AMP Energy (most varieties) | 500 ml can | 160 |
| Vitaminwater Energy | 500 ml bottle | 82 |
| Jolt Energy | 355 ml can | 140 |
| Black Stallion energy drink | 250 ml can | 80 |
| CAFFEINATED WATERS | | |
| Water Joe | 500 ml | 60 |
| Krank$_2$O | 500 ml | 100 |
| FYXX Hybrid (Original) | 600 ml | 110 |
| Ávitãe | 500 ml | 45 or 90 |
| Element | 500 ml | 50 |

†If the country is not stated, the value is international.

*Range of values from studies in which standard servings of the same beverage were analyzed.

Conversion 355 ml = 12 fl oz. Soda and energy drinks are available in a range of individual serving sizes ranging from 150 ml to 750 ml. This table presents the caffeine content of the smallest commonly available size. The caffeine content of larger sizes can be multiplied up.

**Table 3.2** Caffeine Content of Common Sports Foods, Supplements, and Nonprescription Preparations

| Product | Serving size | Caffeine content (mg) |
|---|---|---|
| SPORTS FOOD | | |
| Powerade Fuel+ sports drink | 300 ml can | 96 |
| PowerBar caffeinated sports gel | 40 g sachet | 25 |
| PowerBar double caffeinated sports gel | 40 g sachet | 50 |
| PowerBar caffeinated gel blasts | 60 g pouch (~9 lollies) | 75 |
| GU caffeinated sports gel | 32 g sachet | 20-40 |
| Carboshotz caffeinated sports gel | 50 g sachet | 80 |
| PB Speed sports gels | 35 g sachet | 40 |
| PowerBar energy bar with ActiCaf | 65 g bar | 50 |
| PREWORKOUT SUPPLEMENTS | | |
| Musashi Reactivate Hardcore | 15 g powder | 120 |
| Body Science (BSc) K-OS | 13 g powder | 150 |
| Jack3d | 5 g powder | Not disclosed on label |
| N.O.-Xplode | 18 g | Not disclosed on label |
| Assault | 20 g | Not disclosed on label |
| 1 MR | 8 g | 300 |
| No-Shotgun | 22 g | Not disclosed on label |
| Amped NOS | 40 g | Not disclosed on label |
| Animal Rage | 1 stick | Not disclosed on label |
| Code Red | 10 g powder | Not disclosed on label |

*(continued)*

**Table 3.2** *(continued)*

| Product | Serving size | Caffeine content (mg) |
|---|---|---|
| ENERGY SHOTS | | |
| V Pocket Rocket | 60 g | 160 |
| Lucozade Alert Plus | 60 g | 120 |
| Ammo Energy | 30 g | 171 |
| Jolt Endurance | 60 g | 200 |
| Original 5-Hour Energy | 60 g | Not disclosed on label but measured as 215* |
| Extra-Strength 5-Hour Energy | 60 g | Not disclosed on label but measured as 242* |
| Decaf 5-Hour Energy | 60 g | 6 |
| FAT-LOSS SUPPLEMENTS | | |
| OxyELITE Pro | 1 capsule | 100 |
| BSc Hydroxyburn Pro | 40 g | 24 mg guarana listed on label |
| BSc Hydroxyburn Hardcore | 1 capsule | 70 |
| Muscle Tech Hydroxycut Hardcore Pro | 40 g sachet | Not disclosed on label |
| Shred Matrix | 1 capsule | Not disclosed on label |
| Animal Cuts | 10 g | Not disclosed on label |
| CHEWING GUMS | | |
| Jolt Caffeine Energy Gum | 1 piece | 33 |
| Military Energy Gum (previously called Stay Alert) | 1 stick | 100 |
| Alert Energy | 1 stick | 40 |
| STIMULANT TABLETS | | |
| NoDoz (USA) | 1 tablet | 200 |
| NoDoz (Australia) | 1 tablet | 100 |
| Excedrin Extra Strength | 1 tablet | 65 |
| OTHER | | |
| Blast Caffeine powder | 1 shake | 100 |

"Not disclosed on label" means that the label notes the presence or addition of guarana, caffeine, 3-methylxanthine, yerba maté, or coffee-bean extract as an ingredient but does not provide information about the dose.

*5-Hour Energy does not disclose proprietary brands, but caffeine levels of these products were measured and reported by Consumer Reports, December 2012.

caffeine content of these products. When no independent information was available, we provided the value reported by the manufacturer. You may have seen tables like this before, perhaps with fewer details or entries. There are some important points to understand when you see information of this type:

- Coffee (particularly commercially brewed) contains highly variable caffeine doses (this variability is described within this chapter).

- Manufacturers do not always accurately report the caffeine content of their products (examples are described within this chapter).
- The caffeine content of foods and beverages may vary from country to country.

# Regulation and Labeling

Caffeine can be a natural ingredient in foods and beverages, including tea, coffee, and guarana. Alternatively, it can be added to foods and drinks during the manufacturing process either as an active ingredient or, more often, on the premise that its bitter taste acts as a distinctive flavoring agent (see Where Does the Caffeine Added to Manufactured Products Come From? and Is Caffeine a Flavoring Agent in Soft Drinks? ). Because caffeine is not considered a nutrient but rather a natural food chemical, it is not always subjected to the same nutrition labeling requirements as other food components. Without accurate, or indeed, any information regarding caffeine content on nutrient information panels, it can be difficult for people to quantify their caffeine intake from these foods. Additionally, when caffeine is found as a natural ingredient of a food product, it is typically not subjected to any regulations regarding limits. In contrast, as a result of safety concerns associated with the addition of caffeine to beverages, the authorities regulating food and drugs in various countries specify maximum (and sometimes minimum) levels of caffeine allowed in certain caffeine-added products along with requirements for labeling.

Internationally, caffeine is typically permitted in caffeine-added drinks at levels ranging from 150 to 400 mg/L. The caffeine content permissible within energy drinks typically exceeds that of cola beverages. The specific food regulations for drinks with added caffeine differ from country to country:

- The Food and Drug Administration (FDA) in the United States limits the amount of caffeine in cola-type beverages to a maximum of 0.02%. This means that the highest level of caffeine allowed in a 355 ml (12 fl oz) can of soft drink is about 72 mg. Below this concentration, the FDA classifies caffeine as *GRAS* (generally recognized as safe). No official limit for caffeine within energy drinks has been established; however, it is considered the drink manufacturer's responsibility to provide a product that is GRAS. For a drink to be considered GRAS, there must be evidence of its safety at the levels used and a basis to conclude that this evidence is generally known and accepted by qualified experts.
- Canadian food regulators limit caffeine in cola-type beverages to levels of 71 mg per 355 ml (12 fl oz), or 200 ppm, and the maximum level of use in all other types of carbonated soft drinks is 53 mg per 355 ml, or

## Where Does the Caffeine Added to Manufactured Products Come From?

We have said that the caffeine content of products such as coffee and tea comes from Mother Nature. But where do food manufacturers get the caffeine that is added to cola drinks, energy drinks, and other human-made products? It depends on the manufacturer and the food regulations of the country involved. Because the chemical structure of caffeine has been identified, chemists could make it in a laboratory, but that rarely has to happen these days. After all, there is a whole industry involved with the decaffeination of coffee and tea products for consumers who want to enjoy the flavor of these beverages or join in the social ritual involved with their consumption without the effects of caffeine. Decaffeination is a complex process that involves steaming the unroasted beans or leaves of the plants and then using solvents to extract the caffeine while leaving the other aromatic and characteristic chemicals intact. The by-product of this industry is large amounts of white crystalline powder—caffeine—that can be added to other products according to food laws.

Some added-caffeine products add naturally occurring caffeine via a less direct route. In other words, the manufactured product may contain guarana, kola nuts, yerba maté, or some other plant compound that is a source of caffeine. Why take this approach? Sometimes the manufacturer tries to market the product as more natural, although this is a technicality because in the end it all boils down to the same old trimethylxanthine (caffeine). In other cases, the manufacturer may be trying to get around food regulations that prevent the addition of caffeine to a food but permit the addition of natural flavorings. Again, this is a technicality, but it can cause some confusion to the consumer, who may not be able to identify the total caffeine content of the product from the information provided on the label.

150 ppm. No formal Canadian regulations for energy drinks have been implemented to date. However, Health Canada's scientific assessment supports the establishment of an initial maximum limit for total caffeine of 400 mg/L with a maximum amount of caffeine not to exceed 180 mg per single-serve container. Health Canada also intends to prohibit the use of caffeinated energy drinks in premixed alcoholic beverages.

- In Australia and New Zealand, the maximum caffeine concentration within cola-type beverages must not exceed 145 mg/kg or about 51 mg per 355 ml (12 fl oz) in cola beverages. Regulations for formulated caffeinated beverages (energy drinks) state that they must contain no less than 145 mg/L and no more than 320 mg/L of caffeine. Most of the available energy drinks contain caffeine at this upper level.

- In Europe and the United Kingdom, the maximum allowable level of caffeine in a beverage is not set. However, the European community has agreed to mandatory labeling of all products containing more than 150 mg of added caffeine per liter. Throughout the European Union, any beverage makers who produce drinks above this concentration must inform consumers of the high caffeine content and provide the exact amount of caffeine on the product label.

Typically, food regulators require all manufacturers adding caffeine to beverages to indicate the presence of caffeine on product packaging. Internationally, once a caffeinated beverage contains in excess of 150 mg/L, the quantity of caffeine is also provided.

When assessing food regulations, we must remember that regulators set caffeine limits in terms of the concentration of caffeine in the product. However, people are typically more interested in the total caffeine dose they consume—after all, this is what leads to the physical and mental effects in the body. The individual dose from a caffeine-containing product can easily be calculated as

$$\text{individual dose} = \text{caffeine concentration} \times \text{volume consumed.}$$

One strategy that drink manufacturers employ to increase the so-called fix associated with their particular beverages is to increase the volume of a single serving. In fact, some energy drinks now come in 750 ml sizes. This translates into a greater dose of caffeine for the consumer while remaining within regulatory requirements. The manufacture of these giant serving sizes (see The Caffeine–Calorie Effect: The Real Sinister Side of Caffeine?) and the combination

## Is Caffeine a Flavoring Agent in Soft Drinks?

Some manufacturers claim that caffeine is added to soft drinks because it is a flavoring agent that is integral to the taste of their product. The truth of these claims was investigated in a 2007 publication by researchers Russell Keast and Lynette Riddell from Deakin University, Australia. These scientists determined the taste sensitivity of 30 young people by investigating their taste threshold limits for caffeine among the common sweeteners found in Coca-Cola. Then they asked the participants to taste a caffeine-free Coca-Cola (control) against a caffeinated Coca-Cola. Twenty-eight of the 30 participants could not determine which test beverage contained caffeine regardless of their individual taste sensitivity to caffeine. The researchers concluded that caffeine is not an important flavoring agent. Rather, its presence is intended to create a buzz for the consumer, lead to beverage addiction, or both!

of caffeine with alcohol in beverages (see The Emergence of CABs) is a pivotal concern for health and regulatory authorities.

Can you trust food manufacturers to produce beverages that comply with the specified caffeine regulations? According to a recent comprehensive review of the caffeine content of national-brand and private-label (store-brand) carbonated beverages, you can. At least, this is the case in the United States and among cola manufacturers. Two American researchers, K. Chou and Leonard Bell, from the University of Auburn, Alabama, analyzed 131 carbonated beverages—typically cola types—purchased from a variety of outlets. They compared them with both the FDA caffeine limit and the manufacturers' claims. Only one of the beverages (Vault Zero = 74 mg per 355 ml [12 fl oz]) was above the 72 mg per 355 ml limit for maximum caffeine content. They also demonstrated a wide range in the caffeine contents across all beverages they tested (from 4.9 to 74 mg per 366 ml). As a result, they suggested that consumers would benefit from caffeine values on food labels.

Typically, most store-brand beverages contained less caffeine than their national-brand counterparts. The national-brand beverages also contained values that reflected the caffeine content specified by their manufacturers. This suggested a high degree of quality control during cola production. This study, along with other smaller studies in various countries, suggests that when caffeine is added during the manufacturing of beverages, the amount of caffeine delivered to consumers can be tightly controlled. It also demonstrates that in the case of carbonated beverages, the differences in caffeine content among beverages and brands are likely to be greater than the differences among the same beverage purchased either on different occasions or from different locations.

A survey of 180 athletes from Ghana in Africa revealed that 62% of athletes reported consuming at least one can of energy drink per week—a prevalence higher than that reported by U.S. college students. The reasons for using energy drinks included replenishing lost energy after training or a competition (54%), providing energy and fluids to the body (26%), improving performance (10%), and reducing fatigue (5%). Marketing truly has an international reach!

*Buxton and Hagan (2012)*

## Dose Variability in Naturally Caffeinated Products

Do coffees from one outlet give you more of a hit than others? Or have you ever experienced a different high from the same coffee purchased on different days? Is it possible that you are getting significantly different caffeine doses? Is this even a problem?

## The Emergence of CABs

In 2010, the U.S. Centers for Disease Control and Prevention (CDC) released a fact sheet on the emerging public health impact of caffeinated alcoholic beverages (CABs). CABs are premixed beverages that combine alcohol, caffeine, and other stimulants. They may be malt- or distilled-spirits-based and usually have higher alcohol content than beer (i.e., 5%-12%). CABs have experienced rapid growth in popularity since being introduced into the U.S. marketplace; for example, according to the CDC report, the two leading brands of CABs together experienced a 67-fold increase in sales! The report highlighted that when alcoholic beverages are mixed with energy drinks, a popular practice among young people, the caffeine in the energy drinks can mask the depressant effects of alcohol. This potentially leads to greater risk-taking behavior. And despite popular belief, caffeine has no effect on the metabolism of alcohol by the liver and thus does not reduce breath alcohol concentrations or reduce the risk of alcohol-related harm. Later in the same year, the FDA warned four companies that the caffeine added to their malt alcoholic beverages was an unsafe food additive and stated that further action, including seizure of their products, was possible under federal law. The interaction between caffeine and alcohol is clearly a public health issue of concern (see chapter 6 for further discussion).

Drinks containing caffeine as a natural component, such as tea and coffee, vary in the caffeine dose they provide. The differences in caffeine content can be explained by many factors, including the species of plant origin and the effects of commercial processing such as the time and conditions of storage and transport. The next major source of variability happens in the hands of the commercial or domestic beverage maker—for example, as a result of the amount of coffee or tea used, the extraction method (e.g., percolated, drip), and the temperature and amount of water used. This natural variability in caffeine content is the reason why food labeling requirements in most countries do not mandate that tea and coffee manufacturers specify the caffeine content of their products.

Are these natural variances large enough to be significant to the consumer or athlete? A number of researchers have quantified the magnitude of the variability in caffeine content of similar tea and coffee beverages. Their findings are surprising—and concerning.

- Researchers from the University of Florida at Gainesville quantified the caffeine content of 20 specialty coffees (including more than 7 decaffeinated varieties) purchased from commercial coffee vendors in their local area. They found that the caffeine contents of these coffees varied considerably, with a mean value of 188 mg (standard deviation of 36 mg) and a range of 58 to

259 mg for a 475 ml (16 oz) cup. To add further intrigue, the researchers then purchased the same specialty coffee (Starbucks Breakfast Blend) on six consecutive days from their local outlet. Again, they found a wide range of caffeine concentrations in the same standard brew—from 259 to 564 mg, depending on the day of purchase. The bottom line from this study was that there are substantial differences among types of commercial coffee products and even within different versions of the same standardized retail coffee drink.

- In 2001, the Food Standards Agency (FSA) in the United Kingdom conducted one of the most comprehensive surveys on the caffeine content of hot beverages ever undertaken in a single country. The context was their advice to pregnant women to limit their intake of caffeine to less than 300 mg per day in light of research suggesting that caffeine intakes above this threshold may be associated with low birth weight and, in some cases, miscarriage (see chapter 6 for more information on the safety aspects of caffeine). This warning included information on the number of beverages that equated to 300 mg of caffeine. The recommendations were based on caffeine levels in servings of tea and coffee prepared under laboratory conditions according to standardized procedures. To avoid any inconsistency between the laboratory values and the levels consumed in real life, the FSA then collected 400 samples of teas and coffees prepared by consumers in family homes and workplaces or purchased in retail settings from 10 areas across the United Kingdom. The drinks were analyzed to determine the concentration of caffeine in a serving (i.e., per cup or mug). The primary finding was that there was a large variance in the caffeine content of these beverages. However, for both tea and instant coffee, the highest caffeine dose from any single serving did not exceed 120 mg, suggesting a lower degree of risk associated with overexposure to caffeine from these sources. In contrast, commercial fresh coffee demonstrated broad ranges of caffeine content—from 15 to 254 mg per serving—from the 52 retail samples that were analyzed. The potential exposure to higher levels of caffeine is of greatest concern to anyone who is sensitive to the side effects of caffeine or who wants to consume a small amount of caffeine.

But doesn't this variability simply reflect the various serving sizes of tea and coffee? Correct—in part! The retail coffee samples in both of the studies just described included coffees with significantly different serving volumes, such as espressos, long blacks (talls), lattes, filter coffee, and cappuccino-style coffees. The beverage sizes varied from 30 ml (1 oz) to 475 ml (16 oz). This obviously explains some of the variability in the caffeine content, because vendors typically use more ground coffee when making larger beverages to maintain the palatability and strength of flavor.

So, what happens to caffeine variability when the variety and volume of coffee are more consistent? Between 2006 and 2008, we measured the caffeine content of 133 espresso coffees purchased from commercial outlets in a number of Australian capital cities. Initially, our rationale for collecting espresso coffee was that an espresso shot is the most basic form of coffee drink, limiting many variables such as the addition of significant amounts of milk, water, and sugar. Secondly, the espresso shot often forms the foundation of other types of retail coffee such as lattes and cappuccinos. Therefore, the caffeine dose found in an espresso should be equal to or less than the dose found in the larger coffee varieties.

> I heard that there's a tray of espresso coffees in the tunnel for the England rugby team to down on the way out to the pitch before every game. Does this work? Is coffee the same as caffeine?
>
> *Olympic strength and conditioning coach, multisport*

We collected the coffees from major shopping centers and retail café zones by asking each vendor for a takeaway espresso. If the vendor asked whether we wanted a double shot, we indicated that we wanted only a single shot. If we weren't asked, we did not specify a concentration. We used this standardized approach to ensure that our results would reflect the likely experiences of every-day consumers. We asked each barista about the quantity and type (robusta or arabica) of coffee used and found that the blends were predominantly arabica based. There was a range in the volumes of our samples—from 17 to 87 ml (0.5-3 oz). However, this was far less than the range in previous studies involving

## The Caffeine–Calorie Effect: The Real Sinister Side of Caffeine?

Russell Keast and colleagues from Deakin University recently took their research one big step further. They wanted to assess whether removing caffeine (a bitter flavor) from soft drinks would also allow the removal of sucrose (an antagonistic sweet flavor and source of energy) without affecting the overall flavor of the beverages. Remarkably, they determined that by removing the caffeine from the soft drinks, they could eliminate 10 percent of the sucrose without affecting flavor, which equated to 116 kJ (28 calories) per 500 ml serving. They then did some further calculations and looked at the impact this reduction in energy might have on the obesity levels of a population. By matching the calorie reduction in the drink to the average soft drink consumption of American adults, they determined the reduction would cause a weight loss of 0.6 kg for every U.S. adult! Of course, there's always Coke Zero or Pepsi Max if you want to remove nearly all the calories.

the broader varieties of coffees. The results of our analysis confirmed the earlier findings of a significant variance in the caffeine content of commercial coffee drinks, with a mean value of 108 mg per serving (standard deviation of 37) and a range of 25 to 214 mg. That's an 8.5-fold variance between the least and most concentrated espresso samples! Again, we saw evidence that unsuspecting consumers could be exposed to high caffeine doses.

We have also commenced a study on the variability of caffeine in espresso purchased at the same franchised coffee outlets across different locations. We are comparing both the day-to-day and site-to-site variance in the caffeine content of a standard coffee purchase. Some preliminary results are summarized in table 3.3.

Clearly, large variability in caffeine content is again evident. However, it appears that some larger retail coffee makers (such as Starbucks, Gloria Jean's, and McDonald's) are capable of providing more consistent caffeine doses to their customers compared with other coffee suppliers. We might speculate that the greater consistency is explained by the bulk supply of roasted coffee beans used throughout the multiple outlets operated by these companies. In addition, it is possible that staff receive more detailed training regarding the standardization of beverage preparation. It at least suggests a possibility that commercial coffee operators could produce sufficiently reliable coffee beverages to allow reporting on typical caffeine doses, which would prove useful to many customers. The bottom line for the moment, however, is that there are clear reasons why one coffee may give you more of a buzz than the next!

**Table 3.3**   Caffeine Content of Espresso Coffee Purchased From Various Australian Outlets of the Same Retail Chain (Difference Within the Same Location)

| Coffee chain* | n | Mean (SD) | Range |
|---|---|---|---|
| Coffee Club | 7 | 113 (38) | 82-177 |
| Gloria Jean's | 6 | 145 (11) | 130-162 |
| Muffin Break | 6 | 137 (49) | 68-186 |
| Donut King | 6 | 134 (51) | 82-214 |
| BB's | 5 | 115 (42) | 81-189 |
| Zarraffas | 4 | 62 (11) | 49-75 |
| Starbucks | 4 | 79 (13) | 63-91 |
| McDonald's (Not McCafé) | 4 | 70 (13) | 54-83 |
| Goldstein's | 4 | 91 (27) | 54-114 |

*Data only included for retailers with four or more locations sampled.

# Variability of Cold and Iced Coffee Drinks

The popularity of prepackaged, ready-to-consume, cold coffee beverages has increased dramatically in the past 5 years. Some of these varieties include coffee double shots or guarana as an added ingredient. They are marketed using similar techniques to those employed by energy-drink manufacturers, with the promise of hits, rushes, boosts, or similar euphoric responses. Typically, only those drinks with added guarana are required to specify the caffeine concentration on the nutrition labels.

In 2008, we set out to investigate the caffeine content of these widely consumed beverages within Australia. To do this, we purchased 20 varieties of commercial iced coffee on three separate occasions to ensure that we sampled drinks from different production dates. The caffeine content was analyzed and we calculated the caffeine concentration, caffeine per serving size, and total caffeine in the purchased container. The results are summarized in table 3.4.

We also contacted the drink manufacturers to collect information from them on the caffeine content of their drinks. Some were unable to tell us! We plotted the difference between our findings and the manufacturer's reported caffeine content (see figure 3.1). Our results were similar to the findings for hot coffees. Caffeine concentrations varied greatly among the products, with a mean level of 19 mg per 100 ml (standard deviation = 9) and a range from 7 to 35 mg per 100 ml. Although there was a large difference between drinks, the difference between different samples of the same brand was small, showing good quality control during production. The average caffeine content expressed per carton (~600 ml) was 99 plus or minus 50 mg (range = 33-197 mg per carton). In more than half the brands, the manufacturer underestimated the true caffeine content of the product by more than 10%, highlighting the importance of independent verification of the caffeine content of popular beverages.

Intriguingly, we also discovered that many of these drinks have concentrations of caffeine similar to formulated caffeinated energy drinks—five iced coffees contained $\geq 30$ mg/100 ml of caffeine. Given that these beverages are often sold and consumed in large volumes (typically 500-750 ml), the final result may be a large caffeine dose to consumers. It would appear, then, that the health warnings that are mandatory on energy drinks, such as suggested maximum daily consumption levels, should also be added to some commercial iced coffee drinks. Many people may not consider them to be a potent caffeine source.

**Table 3.4**  Mean, Standard Deviation, and Range of Caffeine Content of Coffee-Flavored Milk Purchased From National Grocery Distributors

| Brand | Mean (mg caffeine/ 100 ml) | SD* | Container volume (ml) | Caffeine (mg/ serving) | Manufacturer's caffeine claim (mg/100 ml) | % difference between actual and manufacturer's claim |
|---|---|---|---|---|---|---|
| Breaka Strong | 32.9 | 0.8 | 600 | 197 | 28 | 17.5 |
| Dare Double Espresso | 35.4 | 1.9 | 500 | 177 | 20 | 77 |
| Ice Break Loaded | 34.4 | 2.0 | 500 | 173 | 32 | 7.5 |
| Rush Intense Coffee | 30.8 | 3.5 | 500 | 154 | 27 | 14 |
| Ice Break | 28.1 | 2.6 | 500 | 141 | 23.2 | 21 |
| Dare Espresso | 24.0 | 2.4 | 500 | 120 | 14 | 71 |
| Farmers Union | 19.1 | 1.2 | 600 | 115 | 18 | 6 |
| Jacaranda | 19.1 | 1.1 | 600 | 115 | 11 | 74 |
| Farmers Union Light [†] | 17.8 | - | 600 | 107 | 18.8 | -5.5 |
| Big M Double Strength | 19.2 | 2.7 | 500 | 96 | 20 | -4 |
| Breaka | 17.1 | 2.7 | 500 | 86 | 14.8 | 15.5 |
| Big M Edge | 17.0 | 0.7 | 500 | 85 | 15 | 13 |
| Breaka Lite | 14.7 | 2.8 | 500 | 74 | 13.1 | 12 |
| Dare Cappuccino | 12.9 | 1.4 | 500 | 64 | 12 | 7.5 |
| Rush Wicked Latte | 12.4 | 1.4 | 500 | 62 | 10 | 24 |
| Rush Mocha Kenya | 12.0 | 0.1 | 500 | 60 | 11 | 9 |
| Dare White Chocolate Mocha | 9.7 | 1.1 | 500 | 49 | N/A | N/A |
| Oak | 12.4 | 0.9 | 300 | 37 | 15 | -17 |
| Woolworth's Iced Coffee | 11.2 | 0.3 | 300 | 34 | N/A | N/A |
| Brownes Cappuccino | 6.6 | 0.4 | 500 | 33 | N/A | N/A |
| **Average (standard deviation)** | **19.3 (8.7)** | | | **99 (50)** | | |

*Indicates SD of samples from one brand across three production dates. N/A indicates not available from manufacturer.

[†]Only purchased on one occasion.

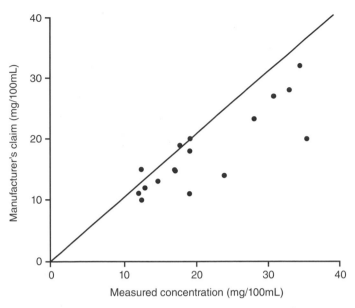

**Figure 3.1** Caffeine content of commercial iced-coffee beverages (manufacturer's claimed value versus independent testing). Line denotes hypothetical manufacturer = independent test (B. Desbrow, unpublished data). Any data point to the right of the line indicates that the manufacturer underreported the actual caffeine content.

Data from B. Desbrow, M. Henry, and P. Scheelings, 2012, "An examination of consumer exposure to caffeine from commercial coffee and coffee flavoured milk: An update," *Journal of Food Composition and Analysis* 28(2): 114-118.

## Is Caffeine a Hook to Develop the Taste for Healthy Foods?

Jennifer Temple and colleagues from the University of Buffalo, New York, have undertaken a number of studies on the effect of caffeine on our liking for beverages, trying to discern how it influences our eating and drinking behavior. A recent study involved subjects drinking a caffeinated or non-caffeinated beverage while trying new types of yogurts with novel and unusual flavors over a four-day period. It found that the liking for these yogurts increased over time, especially when paired with the caffeinated drinks and especially in the case of low-calorie yogurt. The researchers concluded that simultaneous caffeine intake may improve the liking and consumption of novel-flavored foods, particularly if the food is not highly liked to begin with. In fact, they suggested that caffeine pairing may be a way to increase the appetite appeal of other foods with low-energy density such as vegetables and fruit! Looks like caffeine's coercive powers could be used in the fight for nutritional good as well as nutritional evil!

# Is the Caffeine Variance of Coffee Significant for Athletes?

The magnitude of these caffeine differences can be significant for athletes. Let's use Peter to illustrate this. Peter is a 75 kg cyclist who takes his sport seriously and trains 5 days per week. On Saturdays, he stops at his local coffee shop for a quick pick-me-up before his weekly criterium race. Table 3.5 outlines the total and relative (mg/kg) amount of caffeine that Peter could be exposed to based on our data regarding the variability of caffeine doses. The coffees are divided into three categories:

1. Highest 10% caffeine = the range of the highest 10% of caffeine values recorded.
2. Average caffeine dose = the average of all caffeine values recorded.
3. Lowest 10% caffeine = the range of the lowest 10% of caffeine values recorded.

Data are provided for single- or double-strength coffee depending on Peter's personal coffee preference or the barista's generosity and caffeine techniques.

According to this table, we can see that Peter's exposure to caffeine could easily vary by up to 2 mg/kg from just one single-strength coffee hit. Differences in caffeine doses of this magnitude are likely to induce different physical and mental responses in Peter. This isn't the end of the story, however. If Peter's friends Lisa (50 kg) and Stuart (100 kg) join him in this activity, they add the variability of body mass to the variability of caffeine dose. This trio varies in their caffeine exposure from a range that approaches the upper limit of where we now know that caffeine exerts its performance benefits to below the likely performance-enhancing range. Like Goldilocks and her variable experience with

**Table 3.5**  Peter's Potential Differences in Caffeine Exposures From Retail Coffee

| Strength of coffee* | Single | Double | Single | Double |
|---|---|---|---|---|
| | TOTAL CAFFEINE | | RELATIVE CAFFEINE | |
| Highest 10% caffeine | 172-214 | 344-429 | 2.3-2.8 | 4.6-5.7 |
| Average caffeine dose | 106 | 212 | 1.4 | 2.8 |
| Lowest 10% caffeine | 25-68 | 50-137 | 0.3-0.9 | 0.7-1.8 |
| Difference in mean of ranges (highest-lowest) | 146.5 | 293 | 2 | 3.9 |

Values are expressed as total caffeine or relative caffeine (i.e., caffeine per kg body weight).

*Based on espresso data (Desbrow et al. 2007).

porridge, one espresso might have too little caffeine, too much, or just the right amount depending on the coffee and the person who drinks it. This variability in the caffeine content of coffee underlines one difficulty of using this popular beverage as a source of caffeine for performance enhancement (see chapter 9 for further discussion).

> I use sport gels only for the caffeine. I hate them. Makes my face want to screw up when I take them, but I know the caffeine will help me. They're a necessary evil. I only use them in competition.
>
> *Olympic endurance athlete*

We have now clearly demonstrated the difficulty in determining daily caffeine intakes when people consume commercial coffee, whether hot or cold. If you are interested in determining your caffeine intake, the real source of confusion is the within-drink variance—when the same drink varies from day to day or place to place. This variability reduces the confidence that you can accurately quantify the dose of caffeine received when you visit your local café. The caffeine content of other products may be easier to track because you only require a long list of specific caffeine values of individual products (as in the tables in this chapter).

## The Bottom Line

Based on the food regulations in your country, a large number of drinks, foods, supplements, and sport products can be a source of caffeine in your everyday diet or for specific activities. The source of caffeine is typically a leaf, bean, or other part of a plant, but how it got into your drink, food, or supplement can be simple or more complicated. Furthermore, the dose can be quite variable in the case where Mother Nature was mostly involved or more static in the case of mostly human-made products, which are more tightly regulated. Although tables such as the ones provided in this chapter provide a guide to the caffeine content of commonly consumed servings of these products, in some cases the actual caffeine content may be quite different from one serving to another of the same product.

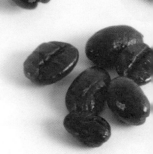

# Chapter
. . . . . . . . . . . . .
# 4

# Caffeine Use in Daily Life

Although this book is about the use of caffeine in sport, we can't just tell the story by leaping to information on caffeinated sport gels or the high-end coffee machines installed in the team buses of professional cycling teams; rather, we need to gather context about caffeine use in our everyday lives. There are two reasons for this. The first is that, as future sections of the book show, when it comes to caffeine use by athletes, the public has strong views that are often confused and confusing. Looking at the typical patterns of caffeine use in the community provides perspective and objectivity to these views. The second reason is to allow athletes who use caffeine to enhance their performance to integrate these strategies into their total daily caffeine intake. Although you might be an athlete for 2 hours and a citizen for the other 22, any caffeine that you consume within a day is the same chemical, chosen for the same reasons (i.e., improving your feelings of well-being and your ability to achieve your chosen activities). It makes sense to choose the caffeine sources and doses that fit with the big picture of your life as well as your sporting goals. This means we need an appreciation of how caffeine has become such a big part of daily life and whether special populations who think they have a particular reason for consuming caffeine treat it differently overall.

Because of its broad social acceptance, low cost, and high availability, more people than ever are regular consumers of caffeine in its various food and beverage forms. It has been suggested that four out of every five people in Western cultures consume caffeine every day. To get a feel for how astonishing this figure is, consider that many people are now more likely to consume caffeine on a daily basis than fruit! Importantly, these high rates of consumption mean that not all athletes who have caffeine in their systems while they train or compete have the intention of gaining a performance advantage. Indeed, some athletes may compete without even realizing they have consumed caffeinated products! As a result, when caffeine is prohibited by antidoping codes, it is subject to threshold (cutoff) limits that attempt to distinguish between habitual caffeine use and deliberate use for sports performance. Chapter 7 provides an overview of the changing status of caffeine in antidoping programs.

It is hard to get figures for the typical caffeine consumption of the average person. The most commonly cited figures for caffeine intake in various countries come from food balance data collected in 1995 (see table 4.1), in which apparent food availability in a country was simply divided by the number of people in the population to derive an average intake. Several limitations of this methodology stand out, including the inability to account for wastage and the inclusion of nonconsumers within the head count. Additionally, these figures only consider caffeine intake from coffee and tea. Nevertheless, they allow an equal comparison of caffeine intake across various parts of the world. The highest caffeine intakes were found in Scandinavian countries, with mean intakes of 320 to 400 mg or 5 to 6 mg/kg. Meanwhile, very low intakes (>50 mg or 0.5 mg/kg) were recorded in the population hubs of India and China. Intakes in countries such as the United States, United Kingdom, France, Italy, and Australia appear modest, with mean daily caffeine intakes from 170 to 230 mg or 2 to 3 mg/kg, at least from coffee and tea sources. There are some major reasons, however, for thinking that these values underestimate the current caffeine intakes of the general population.

Two key reasons explain the increasing likelihood of more frequent and higher intakes of caffeine. First is our seemingly endless love affair with coffee. This aromatic beverage is so embedded in society that there are now more than 700 coffee apps available on iTunes to point you to the best location, method, or accompaniment for your fix. And of course, every other home now seems to have an espresso machine or coffee-making device, with people undertaking barista courses as a leisure-time activity. The second change is the ever-increasing variety of caffeinated products, many of which could be best described as functional foods (foods that have biological functions outside the direct supply of nutrients). Products in this category include carbonated energy drinks; energy shots; sport gels, drinks, and waters; and chewing gums. These foods and beverages have typically been developed to provide an immediate caffeine zap for those in need.

Let's now take a look at trends in coffee consumption. For this example we will use population trends in Australia, but the same shifts in consumer behavior are evident throughout North America and some European countries. In 1949, every Australian drank 3.2 L of tea a year and 0.2 L of coffee (a hangover of English heritage). In the early 1950s, the cappuccino machine arrived, along with mass immigration from Italy. As far as can be established, the first machine was installed in 1953 at the University Café in Lygon Street, Melbourne. And thus began coffee's conquest of Australia.

By 1979, Australians reached a crossover point where they consumed 1.7 L of tea and 1.7 L of coffee a year. From the perspective of caffeine intake, the swing from tea to coffee is significant because tea typically contains less caffeine than coffee (see chapter 3). The momentum toward coffee didn't end there, however. Today, tea consumption is below 0.8 L and coffee is more than 4 L per person per year. Put another way, in 50 years Australians have changed their weekly intake from two cups of tea to three cups of coffee. Furthermore, market research agency BIS Shrapnel estimates that outside the home, Australians drink 1 billion coffees a year, of which 480 million are cappuccinos. Clearly, what was started by the cafés and further boosted by Starbucks, Gloria Jean's, Hudsons, Second Cup, Tim Hortons, and others has made a huge change to the Australian economy, nutritional and social practices, and caffeine intakes. Figure 4.1 compares rates of coffee consumption from various parts of the world, showing that Scandinavian countries continue to lead the world in this activity.

I take very little caffeine on a daily basis so that I can get a bigger effect from it on race day. However, I take caffeine only for hard races (200 mg about 45 to 60 minutes before the final climb or key moment of the race). If it's an easy stage, I do not take any, but if it's extremely hard, I may take up to 300 mg. If the start of the stage is difficult, I take 100 mg before the start and 200 mg toward the end. On the other hand, if the initial kilometers are easy, I wouldn't take the 100 mg dose until later in the stage. I get a strong effect from caffeine ingestion: I am a very mellow kind of guy, and caffeine turns me on. I get a spark from it, and that's the main advantage. Whatever I take, I don't have any trouble falling asleep at night.

*Road cyclist, time-trial finisher of the Tour de France (once in the top 10 of the general classification), and winner of a one-week World Tour race*

If you need further evidence of the availability (and profitability) of caffeine via coffee, try this little experiment. The next time you visit your local shopping center, count the number of outlets selling fresh coffee. Once you have established this number, compare it with that of any other essential product that you may not be able to live without (say, women's shoes!). We have done this experiment numerous times and the result is always an easy win for the coffee retailer. What's more, although these outlets also sell some food and offer a hangout for catching up with friends, a break from the office, or free Internet to catch up on e-mails, the common denominator for the visit is inevitably the cup of java in one of its many variations and its fancy-named serving sizes.

This shift in consumer behavior is not just about the entire adult population seeking greater caffeine doses. One could argue that the drive to drink more

**Table 4.1** Consumption of Caffeine From Coffee, Tea, Yerba Maté, and Cocoa

| COUNTRY | POPULATION (1995) million | COFFEE CONSUMED kton | kg/person each year | CAFFEINE FROM COFFEE mg/person each day | TEA CONSUMED kton | kg/person each year | CAFFEINE FROM TEA mg/person each day | MATÉ CONSUMED kton | kg/person each year | CAFFEINE FROM MATÉ mg/person each day | COCOA CONSUMED kton | kg/person each year | CAFFEINE FROM COCOA mg/person each day | CAFFEINE FROM ALL THESE SOURCES mg/person each day |
|---|---|---|---|---|---|---|---|---|---|---|---|---|---|---|
| Algeria | 28.11 | 54 | 1.92 | 79 | 4 | 0.12 | 5 | 0.0 | 0.00 | 0 | 4 | 0.14 | 1 | 85 |
| Angola | 10.82 | 1 | 0.09 | 4 | 0 | 0.00 | — | 0.0 | 0.00 | 0 | 0 | 0.00 | 0 | 4 |
| Argentina | 34.77 | 36 | 1.04 | 43 | 1 | 0.02 | 1 | 220.0 | 6.33 | 52 | 29 | 0.83 | 5 | 100 |
| Australia | 17.86 | 88 | 4.93 | 202 | 13 | 0.72 | 29 | 0.1 | 0.01 | 0 | | 0.00 | 0 | 232 |
| Austria | 8.04 | 54 | 6.71 | 276 | 2 | 0.19 | 8 | 0.0 | 0.00 | 0 | 24 | 2.98 | 16 | 300 |
| Brazil | 159.02 | 100 | 0.63 | 26 | 2 | 0.02 | 1 | 191.6 | 1.20 | 10 | 110 | 0.69 | 4 | 40 |
| Canada | 29.40 | 129 | 4.39 | 180 | 13 | 0.44 | 18 | 0.1 | 0.00 | 0 | 62 | 2.11 | 12 | 210 |
| China | 1,220.00 | 53 | 0.04 | 2 | 407 | 0.33 | 14 | 0.0 | 0.00 | 0 | 39 | 0.03 | 0 | 16 |
| Colombia | 35.81 | 110 | 3.07 | 126 | 0 | 0.00 | 0 | 0.0 | 0.00 | 0 | 60 | 1.68 | 9 | 136 |
| Denmark | 5.223 | 45 | 8.62 | 354 | 2 | 0.36 | 15 | 0.0 | 0.00 | 0 | 20 | 3.83 | 21 | 390 |
| Egypt | 62.10 | 7 | 0.11 | 5 | 80 | 1.29 | 53 | 0.0 | 0.00 | 0 | 7 | 0.11 | 1 | 58 |
| Finland | 5.107 | 40 | 7.83 | 322 | 1 | 0.16 | 6 | 0.0 | 0.00 | 0 | 1 | 0.20 | 1 | 329 |
| France | 58.10 | 304 | 5.23 | 215 | 11 | 0.20 | 8 | 0.0 | 0.00 | 0 | 171 | 2.94 | 16 | 239 |
| Germany | 81.59 | 580 | 7.11 | 292 | 18 | 0.22 | 9 | 0.5 | 0.01 | 0 | 181 | 2.22 | 12 | 313 |
| Guatemala | 10.62 | 6 | 0.56 | 23 | 0 | 0.04 | 2 | 0.0 | 0.00 | 0 | 4 | 0.38 | 2 | 27 |
| Honduras | 5.65 | 22 | 3.89 | 160 | 0 | 0.00 | — | 0.0 | 0.00 | 0 | 2 | 0.35 | 2 | 162 |
| Hungary | 10.11 | 34 | 3.36 | 138 | 1 | 0.08 | 3 | 0.0 | 0.00 | 0 | 16 | 1.58 | 9 | 150 |
| India | 929 | 16 | 0.02 | 1 | 589 | 0.63 | 26 | 0.0 | 0.00 | 0 | 8 | 0.01 | 0 | 27 |
| Ireland | 3.55 | 7 | 1.97 | 81 | 11 | 3.10 | 127 | 0.0 | 0.00 | 0 | 3 | 0.85 | 5 | 213 |

| | | | | | | | | | | | | | |
|---|---|---|---|---|---|---|---|---|---|---|---|---|---|
| Italy | 57.20 | 276 | 4.82 | 198 | 5 | 0.08 | 3 | 0.0 | 0.00 | 0 | 82 | 1.43 | 8 | 210 |
| Ivory Coast | 13.69 | 2 | 0.15 | 6 | 0 | 0.03 | 1 | 0.0 | 0.00 | 0 | 32 | 2.34 | 13 | 20 |
| Japan | 125.07 | 362 | 2.89 | 119 | 135 | 1.08 | 44 | 0.0 | 0.00 | 0 | 119 | 0.95 | 5 | 169 |
| Kenya | 27.15 | 5 | 0.18 | 8 | 28 | 1.03 | 42 | 0.0 | 0.00 | 0 | 1 | 0.04 | 0 | 50 |
| Kuwait | 1.69 | 2 | 1.18 | 49 | 5 | 2.72 | 112 | 0.0 | 0.00 | 0 | 4 | 2.37 | 13 | 173 |
| Malaysia | 20.14 | 24 | 1.19 | 49 | 13 | 0.67 | 27 | 0.0 | 0.00 | 0 | 16 | 0.79 | 4 | 81 |
| Netherlands | 15.48 | 139 | 8.98 | 369 | 14 | 0.93 | 38 | 0.0 | 0.00 | 0 | 18 | 1.16 | 6 | 414 |
| Nicaragua | 4.12 | 22 | 5.34 | 219 | 0 | 0.00 | - | 0.0 | 0.00 | 0 | 1 | 0.24 | 1 | 221 |
| Nigeria | 111.72 | 4 | 0.04 | 1 | 5 | 0.04 | 2 | 0.0 | 0.00 | 0 | 14 | 0.13 | 1 | 4 |
| Norway | 4.33 | 40 | 9.23 | 379 | 1 | 0.18 | 8 | 0.0 | 0.00 | 0 | 10 | 2.31 | 13 | 400 |
| Paraguay | 4.83 | 6 | 1.24 | 51 | 0 | 0.02 | 1 | 59.2 | 12.26 | 101 | 3 | 0.62 | 3 | 156 |
| Poland | 38.56 | 94 | 2.44 | 100 | 31 | 0.81 | 33 | 0.0 | 0.00 | 0 | 54 | 1.40 | 8 | 141 |
| Russian Fed | 148.46 | 94 | 0.63 | 26 | 143 | 0.96 | 40 | 0.0 | 0.00 | 0 | 182 | 1.23 | 7 | 72 |
| Saudi Arabia | 18.26 | 6 | 0.33 | 14 | 6 | 0.32 | 13 | 0.0 | 0.00 | 0 | 5 | 0.27 | 2 | 28 |
| South Africa | 41.46 | 15 | 0.36 | 15 | 24 | 0.57 | 23 | 0.0 | 0.00 | 0 | 10 | 0.24 | 1 | 40 |
| Sweden | 8.79 | 83 | 9.44 | 388 | 3 | 0.28 | 12 | 0.0 | 0.00 | 0 | 11 | 1.25 | 7 | 407 |
| Switzerland | 7.17 | 48 | 6.70 | 275 | 2 | 0.28 | 11 | 0.0 | 0.00 | 0 | 1 | 0.14 | 1 | 288 |
| Syria | 14.21 | 12 | 0.84 | 35 | 23 | 1.62 | 67 | 8.0 | 0.56 | 5 | 6 | 0.42 | 2 | 108 |
| Tanzania | 30.03 | 2 | 0.07 | 3 | 3 | 0.10 | 4 | 0.0 | 0.00 | 0 | 0 | 0.00 | 0 | 7 |
| United Arab Emirates | 2.21 | 4 | 1.81 | 74 | 5 | 2.13 | 87 | 0.0 | 0.00 | 0 | 2 | 0.90 | 5 | 167 |
| United Kingdom | 58.30 | 131 | 2.25 | 92 | 137 | 2.34 | 96 | 0.0 | 0.00 | 0 | 147 | 2.52 | 14 | 202 |
| United States | 267.12 | 931 | 3.49 | 143 | 80 | 0.30 | 12 | 0.4 | 0.00 | 0 | 596 | 2.23 | 12 | 168 |
| Venezuela | 21.84 | 72 | 3.30 | 135 | 0 | 0.00 | 0 | 0.0 | 0.00 | 0 | 14 | 0.64 | 4 | 139 |

Adapted, with permission, from B.B. Fredholm, K. Battig, J. Holmén, et al., 1999, "Actions of caffeine in the brain with special reference to factors that contribute to its widespread use," *Pharmacological Reviews* 51(1): 83-133.

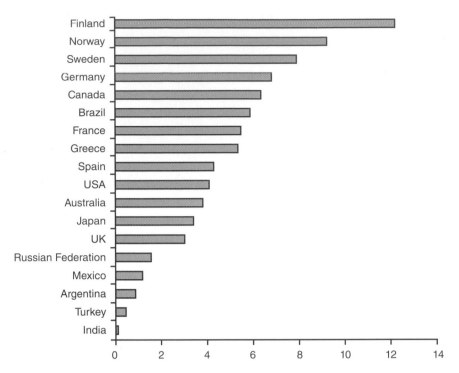

**Figure 4.1**   Current (2010) coffee consumption around the world (annual consumption in kilograms per person).

Data from International Coffee Organization, 2011, Country datasheets. [Online]. Available: www.ico.org/profiles_e.asp?section=Statistics [March 19, 2013].

coffee is underpinned by strong social and marketing movements, along with improvements in the quality and variety of coffees available to drinkers. These factors appeal equally to all demographics. One could therefore speculate that coffee is consumed as much for the social adhesiveness it provides—the way it brings people together—as it is for the flavor and euphoria it produces for the consumer.

Unlike coffee, however, many of the newer functional foods containing caffeine are typically consumed for the sole purpose of making the consumer feel different—providing a jolt, buzz, hit, or added wings! These products are typically marketed directly for this effect and the major customer groups are young people, workers in stressful or physically demanding jobs, and athletes. Typically, their consumption is not linked to social interaction—except at parties!

Let's take the example of the most popular energy drink on the planet—Red Bull. Originating in Thailand in the 1970s, the earliest version was used by truck drivers and laborers to stave off fatigue. Chaleo Yoovidhya, the Thai businessman who invented the drink, then joined with Austrian entrepreneur Dietrich Mateschitz to produce the drink we know today. Red Bull was launched in Austria in 1987 and only entered the U.S. market in 1997. Its market growth

## Does Energy-Drink Marketing Work?

Brenda Malinauskas and her colleagues from East Carolina University in North Carolina conducted a study to determine patterns of energy-drink consumption among college students. They examined the frequency of energy-drink use associated with six purposes—to stay awake or allow sleep deprivation, to increase energy in general, to help while studying, to help when driving for long periods of time, to drink with alcohol while partying, and to treat hangovers. In an average month in the semester, 51% of the nearly 500 participants reported consuming at least one energy drink. The majority of users consumed energy drinks to stay awake (67%), to increase energy (65%), and to drink with alcohol while partying (54%). The majority of users consumed only one energy drink to deal with most situations, although when combined with alcohol intake and partying, it was common practice to consume three or more energy drinks (49%).

could only be described as astronomical, and today the company sells more than 4 billion cans worldwide. Red Bull is so confident in its brand that it launched a cola product (Red Bull Cola) in 2008 to compete against the established cola giants. Of course, in a counterattack the cola giants have released their own energy drinks and have exploited many of the same marketing strategies used so successfully by Red Bull—a whole new cola war!

Regardless of the brand, the popularity of energy drinks has irreversibly forged new ways in which we can consume caffeine. Additionally, their aggressive marketing strategies are attempting to shift the general consensus on how often one should make use of the benefits of caffeine. For instance, according to Red Bull's promotional material (www.redbull.com), a caffeine-fueled energy boost is useful on the road, during lectures and study sessions, at work, while playing sports, and while going out day and night. This doesn't leave a young person with a great deal of time for a caffeine-free existence!

For the person interested in rapidly or regularly exploiting the effects of caffeine, energy drinks are only one of many alternatives. Energy shots, energy ice blocks, sport gels, sport drinks, sport waters, iced coffee beverages with added guarana, chewing gums, caffeinated alcoholic beverages, and nasal sprays containing caffeine have all been developed in the past 10 to 15 years. Like energy drinks, they are marketed primarily to younger adults.

Whether it can be explained by people's shift to coffee, the popularity of the new trend in iced coffee, or perhaps the buzz from the latest energy drink, the bottom line has been a substantial increase in everyday caffeine intake. This is particularly the case among younger people, whose traditional caffeine intakes have been lower than those of adults. The changes in the food supply and the

## Caffeine: Something in the Air?

Is it old-fashioned to consume something by mouth? AeroShot Pure Energy would make you think so. This product presents a new source of caffeine, claiming a "patented delivery system designed to work and work fast." The lipstick-sized canister is placed inside the mouth to deliver a blend of 100 mg of caffeine and B vitamins. Its marketing push describes "No calories. No liquid. No limits."

Aggressive advertising in magazines and college campuses has caused some pushback by scientists. Professor Terry Graham, renowned Canadian researcher of caffeine and coffee, was quick to express concern, saying that unlike coffee, which is absorbed slowly and then taken to the liver for dilution into the bloodstream, an inhalable form of caffeine would lead to rapid absorption from the lungs into blood going straight to the heart. The response from the company is that the inhalable shot of powder actually dissolves in the mouth rather than going to the lungs. They claim that it isn't absorbed any faster than liquid forms of caffeine but represents instead a more practical form of ingestion. In any case, AeroShot is being examined by the FDA.

Another commercially available caffeine spray, Turbo Snort, claims to deliver caffeine nasally for direct delivery to the brain. The spray claims to deliver 1 mg of caffeine per metered spray. There are no published studies of the effectiveness of this product, but caffeine delivered to the brain still needs to be taken into the blood first. The most important clue is available on the label, which states that it is a homeopathic product. Homeopathy is a branch of alternative medicine based on the theory that diseases can be cured with minute doses of drugs that have been diluted to the point that they are almost undetectable. This view is not considered to be evidence based.

cultural norms around caffeine behavior have created a number of issues highlighted by health professionals who have become concerned by the impact of such sustained caffeine exposure:

- As food manufacturers seek new ways to differentiate their products from the rest, where will the love affair with new products and caffeine end? Caffeinated bread? "Smart fish" with omega-3 fatty acids and caffeine for brain function? Caffeinated breakfast cereal to enhance concentration in the classroom?

- Will (or has) the population become inadvertently addicted to caffeine? See the sidebar on addiction (Do I Have a Caffeine Addiction?) for more information.

- Are there any health risks of higher doses of caffeine or longer exposure to caffeine over a lifetime? This issue will be explored in chapter 6.

## Do I Have a Caffeine Addiction?

People often ask if their frequent intake of coffee or energy drinks equates to a caffeine addiction. Psychologists have a system of criteria to define an addiction or dependence (called the *DSM-IV criteria*). To meet this definition, you would need to meet three or more of the following dependence criteria:

1. Tolerance—you need more to get the same hit, or the same amount just isn't working.
2. Symptoms of withdrawal—you don't feel yourself without it, or if you take it the symptoms disappear.
3. The substance is often taken in larger amounts or over a longer period than was intended.
4. Persistent desire—you want it badly!
5. You spend a great deal of time in activities necessary to obtain the substance (e.g., visiting multiple sites or driving long distances)—it's starting to affect your life.
6. Important social, occupational, or recreational activities are given up or reduced because of substance use—it's really affecting your life.
7. Continued use despite knowledge of the dependency—you can't help it!

See your doctor if this sounds like you!

# Use by Special Populations

Concentrating on your office computer is important (just ask your boss). But what if concentrating at work could mean the difference between saving someone's life or not—or even ensuring your own survival? The potential of caffeine to keep you awake, focused, and physically capable now becomes critical. It's for this reason that a significant amount of the knowledge we have gained about the influence of caffeine on cognitive function and exercise capacity comes from research trials funded by military agencies. In many situations, military personnel are athletes whose performance can mean life and death.

It is also through an association with the armed forces that products such as a caffeinated gum were developed to provide a convenient and rapid source of caffeine in operational environments. The manufacture, marketing, and testimonials regarding the use of this supplement speak to the priorities and demands of populations who are routinely exposed to sleep deprivation, danger, and the need to make quick decisions.

Three recent studies have looked at dietary supplements, including caffeine intake patterns, among active personnel in the U.S. and British armed forces.

Christopher Boos and colleagues (2011) collected data on 87 soldiers serving in Afghanistan and compared them with the results of a much larger trial of more than 1,000 soldiers who had been surveyed 2 years earlier while undertaking operations in Iraq. Male soldiers made up a substantial (about 90%) proportion of each study group. The surveys found that the habitual caffeine intakes reported by a substantial minority were excessive. For example, 38% of soldiers drank more than 6 cups of caffeinated drinks each day. This is above the upper sensible limit of daily caffeine intake, generally set at 5 mg/kg or 300 mg (about 5 cups of caffeinated drinks). Around 15% of participants also admitted to the use of stimulants while on deployment, which commonly included caffeine. The authors highlighted that the combination of excessive habitual caffeine intake and use of other stimulants was potentially concerning because it increased the likelihood of caffeine toxicity and adverse effects such as insomnia, irritability, and psychosis.

Meanwhile, the Walter Reed Army Institute of Research analyzed data collected by Joint Mental Health Advisory Team 7 to Operation Enduring Freedom in Afghanistan in 2010. The analysis showed that 45% of deployed service members consumed at least one energy drink daily, with 14% drinking three or more a day. The age or rank of the service members did not contribute to their habitual patterns of use of energy drinks. Service members drinking three or

---

### Staying Alert to Stay Alive in War

Being sleep deprived and fatigued from heavy physical exertion is an occupational hazard for people in the military, with important consequences to health and safety. Tales from the battlefield involving the use of caffeine are legendary and include the chewing of freeze dried coffee grounds. After all, it isn't always practical to stop for a brew or to find a Starbucks in the heat of the moment. Even energy drinks, the caffeine choice du jour for the demographic who make up the bulk of the military, aren't always useful in the field, since the weight and bulk of a liquid reduce their appeal for the MREs (Meals Ready to Eat) that accompany soldiers to war. Within the combat feeding centers, new ideas for adding caffeine to foods such as bars, beef jerky, or trail mix have been tossed around or tried.

In 1999, caffeinated chewing gum caught the attention of military researchers and commanders, and U.S. Congress funded research to determine its effectiveness on military performance. Information provided by the Human Performance Research Center, an education initiative of the U.S. Department of Defense summarizes the following details (http://hprc-online.org/dietary-supplements/ hprc-articles/can-caffeine-chewing-gum-effectively-enhance-warfighter-performance#research-summary):

- A decade of research on caffeinated gum has shown it to be an effective aid to boost the physical and mental performance of military personnel battling fatigue and sleep deprivation. Its effects include maintained reaction times, vigilance, cognitive performance, and enhanced physical endurance.

- Caffeine delivered through chewing gum is absorbed (through buccal mucosa) more rapidly (five minutes) than caffeine delivered in pill or beverage forms (30-45 minutes) and thus counters fatigue more quickly. Other benefits of using caffeinated gum include ease of use, accuracy of dosing, portability, and the gum's ability to withstand extreme temperatures.

- The Committee on Military Nutrition Research (CMNR) has concluded that use of caffeinated gum poses no serious risks to military personnel who may need to use caffeine to fulfill duties. However, caffeine use in extreme environments should be closely monitored to prevent dehydration, and service members in their first trimester of pregnancy face some risk.

- The CMNR provides detailed recommendations on protocols for gum use based on type of performance (physical, mental, and combinations of both) with general recognition that caffeine in doses of 100–600 mg may be used to maintain cognitive performance, reaction speed, and visual and auditory vigilance, particularly in situations of sleep deprivation. A similar dose range (200–600 mg) of caffeine is also effective to enhance physical endurance and may be especially useful to restore some of the physical endurance lost at high altitude. A maximum dose of 1000 mg in a 24-hour period should not be exceeded

- Caffeine has long been a staple of the armed forces to combat fatigue. In 1832, coffee was traded out for rum and whiskey allowances and has been part of army rations ever since. The current First Strike Rations® include caffeinated gum in army supply channels.

The commercial gum, trialed and tested for use with military forces and security personnel and made under authorization of Wrigley's Gum, was initially sold as Stay Alert (NSN #8925-01-530-1219). In 2013 it changed its name to Military Energy Gum. Although it has quickly made its way into civilian markets, testimonials from the company website speak clearly to its use within military environments (www.militaryenergygum.com/testimonials/):

- "This will be sent to me at Fob Endurance. I am deployed to Iraq. This product is a life saver, literally…it just sucks when we all run out."

- "Spent 12 ½ months in Iraq, your gum saved me a few times. Great stuff. I will distribute to my firemen and other first responders."

- "Outstanding product. I am a WWII retired major; former POW. Wish we had this product in WWII. We went days without sleep. We aged fast, and suffered. Thanks for supporting our troops."

more energy drinks a day were significantly more likely to report sleeping an average of less than 4 hours a night than those consuming two drinks or fewer. They were also likely to report sleep disruption related to stress and illness and were more likely to fall asleep during briefings or on guard duty.

Finally, the use of dietary supplements within the American military has been examined by Harris Lieberman and colleagues (2010) from the U.S. Army Research Institute of Environmental Medicine in Massachusetts. This research group surveyed 990 soldiers randomly selected from 11 army bases around the globe. Approximately 12% of respondents reported using dietary supplements from the category *other*, which included caffeine tablets, glucosamine, fish oil, and melatonin. The researchers concluded that compared with civilians, U.S. soldiers use more dietary supplements purported to enhance performance. They speculated that these differences may reflect the unique occupational demands and stresses of military service.

Overall, the studies of caffeine use in the military show a number of key findings:

- The habitual caffeine intake of many soldiers is high.
- Additional caffeine intake may come from other supplements and may be combined with other stimulants.
- Those responsible for the health and well-being of soldiers should try to develop protocols for safe and effective use of caffeine to combat the occupational hazards of their work.
- There is a need for education to integrate the use of caffeine within combat and non-combat elements of the work of the military.

Many other professions place their workers under significant mental and physical stress. For example, firefighters, police and ambulance officers, and staff in hospital emergency departments all undertake highly demanding tasks, often within the framework of shift work or lengthy shifts that affect sleep and arousal. Members of these professions have well-known caffeine habits. But does caffeine improve their ability to do their jobs? Many studies have been conducted to address this question.

Cochrane Reviews extract the results of a group of studies to systematically arrive at a bottom line. One such recently conducted review set out to answer the question, "Is caffeine useful for the prevention of injuries and errors in shift workers?", from the observations collected in 13 separate studies. Unfortunately, none measured an injury outcome. Two trials measured error, and the remaining trials used neuropsychological tests to assess cognitive performance. The trials assessing the impact on errors found that caffeine reduced the number of errors compared with a placebo. One trial comparing the effects of caffeine with a nap found that significantly fewer errors were made in the caffeine group. Other trials comparing caffeine with interventions known to help with sleep issues (e.g., naps, bright light, modafinil) found them to be equally as effective. Based on this evidence, the authors concluded that there was no reason for healthy people who already use caffeine within recommended levels to improve their alertness to stop doing so.

---

### Coffee: The Driver Reviver

How effective are the driver-reviver stops that encourage drivers to take a break when undertaking long-distance driving? A recent study from the Netherlands carefully examined the effects of 1 cup of coffee (80 mg caffeine) on monotonous simulated highway driving in non-sleep-deprived individuals. Participants were asked to drive for 2 hours on a computer simulator, followed by a 15-minute break with or without consuming caffeinated coffee, then a further 2 hours of driving. The results showed that when participants consumed the coffee, they improved their ability to drive as shown by their ability keep the vehicle steady within the lane, the consistency of their speed, their subjective tiredness, and the mental effort required for driving. What isn't yet clear is the effect of a coffee and a muffin!

---

## Use by Athletes

Just how often is caffeine used for its real or believed effects on sports performance? The caffeine habits of athletes have been investigated across a variety of settings, but some care is needed to interpret the findings. This is because most studies ask athletes to fill out a questionnaire designed to assess usual or total dietary practices rather than the prevalence of their caffeine use and the reasons that underpin it. The typical outcome is a description of the athletes' habitual caffeine intake rather than a targeted insight into their use of caffeine for performance enhancement. Furthermore, this approach relies on the honesty and memory recall of the participant. We've tried to focus here on caffeine use by athletes to improve their sports performance, but we admit this is not always possible.

In 1993, Professor Terry Graham, a prolific caffeine researcher from the University of Guelph, Canada, published a study in which 27% of Canadian teenagers reported using caffeine to directly improve their sporting performances. Ten years later, Dr. Gary Slater and his colleagues from the Singapore Sports Council demonstrated a high prevalence of caffeine use (37%) in a group of 160 elite Singaporean athletes across a variety of sports. In 2004, a research team headed by Kathryn Froiland from the University of Nebraska at Lincoln reported lower rates of caffeine consumption following a survey of more than 200 male and female college athletes from one Division I university (11% of all athletes, with a particularly high rate among wrestlers). A year later, similarly low rates of caffeine consumption were observed in a study on Canadian varsity athletes by Kristiansen and colleagues. The authors noted that although caffeine was often consumed, it was for pleasure and alertness rather than its ergogenic benefits. Most recently, in 2010, Dr. Ben Dascombe and colleagues conducted a study on the general nutritional supplement practices of scholarship holders attending the Western Australian Institute of Sport, an elite sport academy. They found that 16 of 72 athletes (22%) reported caffeine use associated with their sport and that male athletes were more likely to report ergogenic caffeine use (31%) compared with female athletes (14%).

> I take 50 to 75 mg of caffeine 45 minutes before the start of competition. On the bike, I take another 50 to 100 mg, usually by means of caffeinated gels. During the run leg of the race I also take 50 to 100 mg in the form of gels, and I suppose I get an additional amount with the Coca-Cola I sometimes drink in some drink stations. I prefer to spread my caffeine intake over the duration of the competition, because I don't like the effect of ingesting it all at once. I get all shaky and have difficulties concentrating.
>
> *Male triathlete, two-time Olympian, winner of five Ironman events*

Taken collectively, these studies indicate that caffeine is consumed for somewhat sport-specific purposes, it is being used by approximately one in four athletes, and its popularity as a potential performance enhancer appears to be static. Two key issues, however, affect the ability of these studies to account for the current caffeine habits of athletes. First, these investigations rely on self-reported information from athletes, which is subject to honesty and memory. Ideally, such data would be confirmed by objective measurements such as plasma or urinary caffeine tests or independent surveillance. Second, the publication date of the research is important. Much of the data on the prevalence of caffeine use by athletes were collected during the 1990s, or more precisely, before January 1, 2004. As will be discussed in chapter 7, on this date there was a big change to the status of caffeine in major antidoping programs. It would be reasonable to expect differences in the behavior (or admitted behavior) of athletes regarding caffeine use before and after this point. This could be a product of nonuse or low use during times when caffeine was considered a prohibited or restricted substance in IOC- and WADA-sanctioned competitions, followed by liberation of intake once caffeine was removed from the list of prohibited substances. Or, it could be the same actual use masked by a deliberate underreporting of intake before the changeover date.

Six newer studies provide a clearer picture of ergogenic caffeine use by athletes in the eras before and after the reorganization of the WADA list. These studies are special for several reasons. In particular, each focused exclusively on caffeine intake by athletes rather than finding it among a number of other items of interest. And, importantly, four involved objective rather than self-reported measures of caffeine intake.

The first report of interest comes from our own research group. It involves a study of caffeine use by a specific group of ultraendurance athletes competing at a major international event about 18 months after the status of caffeine changed on the WADA list. In the study, 140 triathletes from 15 countries, including elite and age-group participants from the 2005 Ironman Triathlon in Hawaii, agreed to complete a prerace caffeine-related questionnaire. The questionnaire investigated their caffeine-related knowledge, sources of caffeine information, experiences using caffeine, and plans for caffeine use throughout the upcoming race. While they completed the questionnaire we also asked if they would consent to giving a blood sample immediately after race completion for quantification of their plasma caffeine level.

A large proportion (73%) of these athletes believed caffeine was ergogenic to their endurance performance, and 84% believed it improved their concentration during an event. The most commonly reported positive caffeine experiences related to the within-competition use of cola drinks (65%) and caffeinated gels (24%). The most popular sources of caffeine information were self-experimentation (16%), fellow athletes (15%), magazines (13%), and journal articles (12%). Not surprisingly, then, our results also indicated that 124 athletes (89%) reported that they planned on using a caffeinated substance throughout the event. However, of more concern was that over one-quarter of the athletes remained either confused or uninformed about the legality of caffeine in sport. Postrace plasma samples ($n = 48$) demonstrated detectable levels of circulating caffeine in all subjects, with mean

> Yeah, the best sports drink in the world is Coca-Cola! Ha-ha! I discovered that when I was suffering out on the lava fields in Hawaii. You know one of the hottest triathlon events you can do on the planet and probably the toughest race. I grabbed the coke at one of the A stations because I was in a bad way. I took a sip and it was like instant energy. I was like, MAN, what do they put in this stuff! It has become a key component of mine in my nutritional plan since that day on. I don't think they designed it for athletes, but it works when you're depleted of sugars. When it gets really tough, my secret weapon is either a Coca-Cola or Red Bull. The mix of simple sugars and caffeine give me the jolt I need.
>
> *Chris McCormack, winner of the 2007 and 2010 Ironman World Championships (Vail, 2012)*
>
> Reproduced by permission.

values of ~4 µg/L or a dose equivalent to ≥3 mg/kg BW. This is similar to the lower ranges of doses that have been shown to improve endurance performance in controlled trials (see chapter 5).

We also demonstrated that the athletes' awareness of antidoping rules regarding caffeine was associated with their actual caffeine intake. Specifically, the dose of caffeine was higher if an athlete was aware that caffeine is an unrestricted substance—about 222 mg in those unaware of the 2004 decision versus 415 mg in those who were aware of the change in the status of caffeine on the WADA antidoping list.

In 2008, two studies highlighted the use of caffeine by high-level athletes across a range of sports in the United Kingdom and Canada. Neil Chester and Nick Wojek from Liverpool John Moores University investigated the caffeine-related behaviors of a large group of cyclists ($n$ = 287) and track and field athletes ($n$ = 193) using a web-based questionnaire. Their participant pool included both elite and well-trained athletes throughout England, Scotland, Wales, and Northern Ireland. Results revealed that among these athletes, the intention to use (attitude) and use of (behavior) caffeine as an ergogenic aid was high. Approximately 2 in 3 cyclists and 1 in 3 field athletes reported consuming caffeine to specifically enhance performance. The practice of consuming caffeine to improve performance was more likely in elite rather than subelite athletes from both sports. The survey also investigated the sources of caffeine-containing products used by these athletes. Of all caffeine-containing products used, coffee, energy drinks, pharmaceutical preparations, and caffeinated sport supplements were the most popular.

In contrast to these investigations, a study of elite Canadian athletes reported modest caffeine use—at least during training phases. Jasmine Tunnicliffe and colleagues from the University of Calgary asked 270 national- and international-level athletes from a range of sports (both summer and winter) to record their food and fluid intake for 3 days, including 2 days of training and 1 day of rest. They subsequently analyzed the dietary records using standardized caffeine values to calculate both the total coffee and caffeine intakes. They found that 33% of the athletes did not report ingesting caffeine in any form, 37% ingested daily intakes of 0 to 1 mg/kg, 23% ingested 1 to 3 mg/kg, 5% reported average caffeine intakes of 3 to 5 mg/kg, and only 2% consumed >6 mg/kg. The researchers concluded that the majority (70%) of high-level Canadian athletes consume dietary caffeine at levels insufficient to elicit performance enhancement, whether or not that is the intention. No differences were noted for caffeine intake between summer and winter sport competitors.

Another insight into caffeine use by athletes in competitions comes from the analysis of urine collected at postevent doping control stations. In chapter 7, we will explore further the circumstances that led to caffeine being placed on, and then removed from, antidoping prohibited lists. One outcome of the 2004 changeover, however, was the addition of caffeine to the WADA Monitoring Program. This means that some urine samples collected at in-competition testing continue to be analyzed for caffeine content with the intention to look for trends in use and potential abuse by athletes. This could be considered objective information about caffeine use rather than relying on athlete self-reports, although we need to take into account a few limitations. These include the selection of athletes to be drug tested

> We've done a lot of studies over the years looking at the effect of sports drinks on endurance performance. We changed the carbohydrate concentrations of drinks and the types of sugar blends with very little effect on the outcomes. The only thing that really seemed to make a difference to performance—at least in lab studies—was the addition of caffeine to the sports drink. Much to our surprise, it seemed to work by maintaining quadriceps strength, which would explain improvements in high-intensity cycling performance.
>
> *Sports scientist and researcher*

in the first place and the limitation of urinary caffeine content as a measure of recent caffeine intake (see chapter 2). Nevertheless, these data are particularly interesting when they are compared over time or between athletes in different sports or levels of competition. If the use of caffeine by athletes is increasing, these data will surely hold the answer.

In order to understand any trend, we first need to set our baseline. That is, what was the use of caffeine before its removal from the WADA list of prohibited substances? In 2005, Dr. Wim van Thuyne and colleagues from an accredited testing laboratory in Ghent, Belgium, published their findings from 11,361 in-competition urine tests collected from 1993 to 2002 across a selection of team and individual sports. Figure 4.2 summarizes urinary caffeine levels from sports in which more than 200 samples were selected. Notwithstanding the limitations of urinary caffeine concentrations as a measure of recent caffeine intake, the study shows evidence of wide variation within sports as well as in apparent caffeine use between sports. Differences between sports included larger numbers of athletes without detectable levels of caffeine in urine in athletics, swimming, and basketball. Conversely, higher average urinary caffeine levels were detected in samples provided by cyclists and bodybuilders. This study further reported that of the 16 athletes who recorded urinary caffeine levels above the permitted threshold of 12 µg/ml, 4 were cyclists and 7 were in strength sports (bodybuilding, weightlifting, and powerlifting).

The next step is to compare our baseline information with reliable follow-up data.

A further study from this group, published in 2006, compared 4,633 samples collected during 2004 with samples taken before the January 1, 2004, change

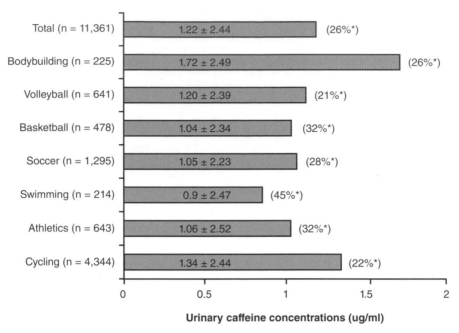

**Figure 4.2** Urinary caffeine concentrations from in-competition testing by an accredited Belgian antidoping laboratory before 2004.

*Number of samples below detection limit.

Adapted from W. Van Thuyne, K. Roels, and F.T. Delbeke, 2005, "Distribution of caffeine levels in urine in different sports in relation to doping control," *International Journal of Sports Medicine* 26(9): 714-718.

to caffeine's antidoping status. Their results indicated that the average urinary caffeine concentration did not change in the 12 months following WADA's decision to remove caffeine from its prohibited substances list. Interestingly, while the overall percentage of urinary caffeine samples greater than 12 μg/ml between the two periods remained the same, the prevalence of these findings in cyclists slightly increased after the removal of caffeine from the list of prohibited substances. This suggests a possible increase in the popularity of caffeine or its dosing protocols among this group of athletes. However, given the short period of time in which the samples were collected following the change in prohibition status, this can only be considered an initial indication.

Recently, Juan Del Coso and colleagues (2011) from the WADA-certified Doping Control Laboratory of Madrid reported on their measures of urinary caffeine in samples received from athletes between 2004 and 2008—more than 20,000 samples! They hypothesized that, due to the liberal use of caffeine in sport during this period, urinary caffeine concentration would increase progressively after 2004. Table 4.2 provides a summary of their data.

These figures regarding caffeine use in competitions from 2004 to 2008 are similar to those obtained when caffeine was banned and thus have not increased, at least in terms of the caffeine doses that athletes are consuming. Furthermore,

**Table 4.2** Urinary Caffeine Concentrations From In-Competition Samples Collected From Athletes Across a Range of Sports After 2004, Analyzed by an Accredited Spanish Antidoping Laboratory

| Year | No. of samples tested | Mean (± SD) urinary caffeine concentrations (µg/ml) | Percentage of samples below detectable urinary caffeine content |
|---|---|---|---|
| 2004 | 3,262 | 1.6 ± 2.3 | 28 |
| 2005 | 4,911 | 1.4 ± 2.3 | 29 |
| 2006 | 4,710 | 1.3 ± 2.2 | 27 |
| 2007 | 4,960 | 1.5 ± 2.4 | 26 |
| 2008 | 2,843 | 1.5 ± 2.2 | 25 |
| Total | 20,686 | 1.5 ± 2.3 | 26 |

Data from Del Coso et al. 2011

the number of samples exceeding the former WADA cutoff (12 µg/ml) appear to have remained consistently low (<1% of samples) throughout this period. In group sport, it appears that athletes have not changed their within-competition caffeine practices.

But what is happening at the level of individual sport? Figure 4.3 takes the urinary caffeine concentrations from in-competition samples collected from athletes across a range of sports before 2004 (Van Thuyne et al. 2005) and compares them with the most recent data after 2004 (Del Coso et al. 2011).

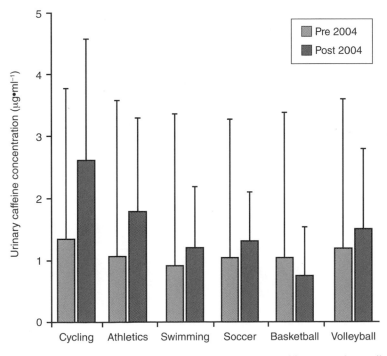

**Figure 4.3**   Urinary caffeine concentrations from in-competition samples collected from athletes before 2004 (Van Thuyne et al. 2005) and after 2004 (Del Coso et al. 2011).

This sport-by-sport analysis suggests trends toward higher uses in endurance sports such as cycling and possibly triathlons (both of which reported significantly higher mean urinary values than any other sports). However, even within these endurance sports where caffeine use is more prevalent, the urinary values still indicate low levels of caffeine consumption by athletes and hence modest within-competition caffeine consumption.

## The Bottom Line

Caffeine is a major part of the daily lives of most people, and over the past decades there have been changes to the amount of caffeine that we consume and the sources that we are likely to get it from. Athletes are both members of the larger community and a special population who might use caffeine for specific purposes. Although there are some problems with getting reliable information on caffeine use by athletes, it appears to be a popular supplement, particularly among competitors in endurance sports. Both the shift in community use of caffeine and the specific change in the position of caffeine in antidoping rules in 2004 may have contributed to the recent changes in the behavior of athletes regarding caffeine use.

Are these changes warranted? We will now take caffeine for a test-drive through the questions we use to judge the suitability of a supplement for use in sport: Is it effective? Is it safe? Is it permissible?

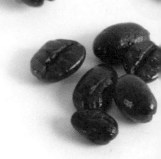

# Chapter

# 5

# Effectiveness

Now that we've established some of the effects of caffeine, it's time to focus on what these might mean in terms of sports performance. As with all potential ergogenic aids, the athlete should work through three levels of consideration: Is it effective? Is it safe? Is it legal? This chapter tackles the question of whether caffeine can truly make an athlete go faster, higher, stronger, or whatever is needed to perform better in sport.

There is a relatively long history of research on caffeine and exercise, and our modern world puts much of it in easy reach of athletes, coaches, trainers, and budding sport scientists. The Internet hosts specialized search engines and databases, such as Google Scholar and PubMed, that can locate studies of interest in a few keystrokes. Popular magazines and websites often repackage the information from such studies, and it also turns up in briefer formats on Facebook and Twitter. We are all for self-learning and the connectivity of the Information Age, but there are some traps involved in converting the results of scientific endeavors into practice in sport. Therefore, in this chapter we not only summarize the current evidence underpinning the effective use of caffeine in sport, but we also pass on some tips to allow you to make sense of future studies.

Our first task is to recognize that not all of the available information on caffeine and exercise is targeted or suited to athletes, and extreme caution may be needed in trying to transfer the results of studies to an athlete's training or competition program. Because caffeine has so many physiological and pharmacological effects, it provides a great opportunity to study metabolism and how remarkable our bodies can be. Exercise adds another component to that story. The good news is that the combination of these elements has drawn the attention of many scientists, making sure the field of caffeine and exercise research is solid and respected. But the trap is that exercise isn't the same as sport, and the context of studies does not always apply to the real-life endeavors of athletes. As a result, some research on caffeine and exercise simply isn't meaningful to athletes

"While I'm racing, caffeine is actually a pretty important part of my day, particularly in the Ironman, where it's such a long race," says Sarah Piampiano, a professional triathlete. She integrates calories and caffeine into her race-day diet using energy gels. Each contains 50 milligrams of caffeine, which Piampiano calls a "shot." "Before the race, I typically take one gel that has one shot of caffeine in it, and then when I get onto the bike, each hour I take one shot of caffeine," explains Piampiano. In the last half of the marathon, she ups her dose to two shots every 20 minutes.

*Murray Carpenter (2012)*

and the results may need to be ignored or heavily filtered to find a practical bottom line. We have seen from the previous chapter that many other people, including the military, firefighters, and manual laborers, undertake exercise as an occupation. So, it's reasonable to expect that some of the available research reflects the specific questions or conditions of these groups rather than athletes.

Every study that sees the light of day in a journal reflects a number of scientific and practical inputs. These include the primary question of interest, the amount of funding available, the availability and limitations of lab equipment and subjects, the technical skill of the scientists, and the degree of focus on measuring mechanisms. And apart from the scientists directly involved in the study, there will be input from the ethics panel that approved the research and other scientists in the peer-review process who helped to shape the final publication. It's hardly surprising that many studies can fall under the technical umbrella of caffeine and exercise.

When we set out to examine the available research on caffeine for sports performance, we decided to narrow our sights to the studies that were most applicable to the interests and activities of athletes. We also identified some key differences in the characteristics of traditional lab-based studies of caffeine and exercise and the features of athletic performance. Table 5.1 at the end of the chapter summarizes these factors to alert readers (and participants) of caffeine research to some caveats that need to be considered when applying the results of caffeine research to the world of sport.

## Does Caffeine Enhance Sports Performance?

In cutting to the chase of whether caffeine can assist sports performance and how to use it to achieve the best outcomes, we have assembled a summary of research on caffeine and sports performance that meets as many of the important features of sport as possible. In particular, we focused on studies involving subjects who were regular participants in sport and undertook specific training programs. In addition, we concentrated on investigations of the effect of caffeine on exercise tasks that resemble sports rather than on studies that simply measured how long a subject could last on a treadmill or lab bike before falling off or nodding off from fatigue or boredom.

We grouped the studies into five categories according to the key characteristics of the sport they best apply to. We summarized the timing and dose of caffeine, and we noted if the caffeine came from a source of special interest, such as from energy drinks and preworkout supplements with other ingredients or from gum so the caffeine is absorbed through the walls of the mouth rather than through the gut. We also looked for other nutritional strategies of interest, such as the intake of carbohydrate during longer sports or the use of other ergogenic aids. Because some readers want the simplest answer possible, we made a judgment call on whether the results of the study show a favorable outcome to real-world sports performance. However, we also added a final column to provide more detail on the actual numbers that determined this outcome, at least in the words of the study report. Some of this information may be more technical than some readers feel comfortable with. Nevertheless, we have included it so that is available for those who are interested.

Because sports differ in what it takes to perform better, we considered it possible that caffeine might work for some sports but not others. And because caffeine has so many actions on the body, we also considered that one type of use (e.g., dose, timing) might attack a specific challenge in some sports but not be suited to others. We noted that because each sport has such specific requirements or practical considerations in terms of the way that drinks and foods can be consumed before, during, or between events, there might be some common ways that caffeine could be used in all sports (e.g., taking it an hour before an event) but also some ways that are unique to an event (e.g., consuming it from supplies at aid stations in a marathon or at halftime in a football match).

Here's how we would sum up our findings in 250 words or less:

- Overall, caffeine seems to be effective in enhancing the performance of most sports, with the greatest effects found in sports that have a strong element of fatigue during or toward the end of the event. The exception to the rule seems to be events of very high intensity or power output lasting seconds, such as sprints or lifts. In these events, caffeine doesn't seem to be consistent in enhancing the outcome of a single effort.

- The typical effective dose of caffeine used in laboratory studies is 5 to 6 mg per kg of the athlete's body weight consumed 1 hour before the event. However, this dose is seen so often in studies simply because scientists often just copy what they know to be successful, even if it is more than is needed or there are alternative ways to do it. What should be more important in real-life sport is finding the smallest dose that achieves the best outcomes and finding various ways that it can be used effectively to suit the specific event or athlete. Newer research shows that in many events and sports, the maximal effective dose of caffeine is about half of the traditionally used level (i.e., 3 mg/kg), and it can be taken at different time points including before the event, spread throughout the event, or toward the end of the event.

- People vary in their response to caffeine, ranging from large positive effects on performance to trivial responses and some negative outcomes.

Of course, athletes want more specific information about caffeine and their sports and events, so following is a more detailed breakdown.

## Endurance Sports

When we speak of endurance sports, we are referring to sustained events lasting more than an hour. Sport scientists have focused most of their research efforts on caffeine and sport on endurance events (table 5.2 at the end of the chapter). Running, cycling, and cross-country skiing challenges have all featured in studies of caffeine supplementation, with the majority taking place in research labs. These lab-based studies provide strong but not unanimous support that caffeine can be beneficial for these activities. Most studies have involved the caffeine supplementation protocol made popular in the 1980s in which athletes consumed a moderate-large dose (5-6 mg/kg) 1 hour before their performance trial. Some studies have commented on the variability of responses within a group of subjects—some people get a large performance boost, some receive a smaller effect, and some even appear to have a minimal or negative experience.

More recent studies have investigated various ways to take caffeine. These show that a variety of caffeine protocols may be useful for endurance sports, including taking it before the event, spreading it out during the event, or a mixture of before and during. Another apparently successful protocol is to hold off on taking caffeine until after the halfway mark of an event, then

I have taken caffeine tablets before games to make me more alert when the ball is bounced. Some players even take them at halftime. It makes your reaction time a little bit better and you feel more alert. It is about finding the right level that suits the individual player. Club doctors always help out in this regard and clearly they would not put their players in jeopardy.

*Shane Crawford, former captain of Australian Football League team (2010)*

rolling it out just before fatigue starts to become apparent. A couple of studies have directly compared a number of caffeine schedules and found them to be equally effective in enhancing performance in an endurance sport. It would appear that, similar to the way we consume caffeine in everyday life, different patterns of intake work for different situations or people.

Similarly, recent investigations have looked at the effectiveness of various doses of caffeine on the performance of endurance sports. Several have shown that relatively low doses of caffeine can enhance prolonged activities. Putting all the studies together, including those that compared a sliding scale of caffeine doses, it appears that intakes as small as 1.5 g/kg (~100 mg) may be beneficial in some circumstances, with the certainty of benefits increasing with increasing doses. However, the improvements top out at a dose of ~3 mg/kg, or 200 to 250 mg in total. This is much lower than the old-fashioned protocols for caffeine use in sport and well within the daily caffeine habits of most adults. It should be stressed that some studies have shown performance impairments when caffeine doses climb above 6 mg/kg, and there is also an increased risk of side effects. So, there is no need to follow the creed of "more is better." Several studies that monitored urine samples at the end of the endurance protocols found that caffeine supplementation can produce performance gains in sport with caffeine concentrations that are well below 12 µg/ml, the threshold previously set by the International Olympic Committee (IOC) as indicative of doping infringement (see chapter 7).

A few investigations of endurance sports have been undertaken in the field during competitions, including cross-country ski races, a half marathon, and an 18 km road race. These studies have been less supportive of performance benefits compared with the laboratory investigations. However, this may be due to other factors in the design, such as small numbers of subjects, caffeine doses at the low end of the apparently effective range, and perhaps the extra variability in conditions that occurs in the real world. We have mentioned that it is difficult to produce exactly the same weather conditions and competitive environment for two or three occasions to allow athletes to truly race the same race in all aspects apart from the use of caffeine. Nevertheless, it is in the real world that athletes need to perform at their best, so it is important to conduct studies in this arena. We challenge sport scientists to do more!

We noted in our summary that at least some lab-based studies have involved conditions that reflect recommended and real-life strategies of athletes—for example, providing subjects with sport drinks or other carbohydrate sources during their time trials and having them eat a carbohydrate-rich meal beforehand. This includes a project we conducted to investigate a practice we saw happening in some endurance sports—cyclists, triathletes, and runners turning to Coca-Cola in the last part of a race in preference to sport drinks. We thought this was a strange choice based on what we knew at the time. However, this was a case when athletes were able to teach us a science lesson (see Does Practice Inform Science, or Does Science Inform Practice?).

Studies of endurance sports have varied according to the dietary conditions under which subjects performed their task—whether they consumed a prerace meal or fasted and whether carbohydrate was consumed during the protocol. We noted in our summary table (5.2) whether researchers allowed their subjects to refuel *during* their performance trial—usually by consuming a sport drink or its equivalent—since this is a key recommendation of sport nutrition guidelines and it appears that caffeine and carbohydrate intake during endurance events influence each other. Researchers from the Georgia Institute of Technology who examined the literature on caffeine supplementation and endurance exercise found some evidence of such an effect. They undertook a meta-analysis, a mathematical approach that combines the results of a body of studies. Their data pooling found that when caffeine and carbohydrate were both consumed during endurance exercise, there was a small benefit to exercise outcomes compared with consuming carbohydrate alone. However, when caffeine supplementation was undertaken in trials in which only water was consumed, there was a twofold larger enhancement of performance than when caffeine was consumed during trials in which subjects also refueled with carbohydrate.

An interaction between carbohydrate and caffeine might be present in several ways. The first idea is that the effects of caffeine are more pronounced in exercise or sporting tasks in which there is a clear case of fatigue and declining performance. The lack of carbohydrate intake during endurance sport would be likely to lead to greater fatigue and thus a greater opportunity for caffeine supplementation to rescue the performance decline. A second idea is that caffeine may increase the ability of the body to deliver the carbohydrate consumed during exercise from the gut to the muscle, increasing its effectiveness as a supplementary fuel source. This may not matter if a large amount of carbohydrate is

They hit 10 kilometers at a fairly brisk 31:15. Shorter was 10 seconds behind Hill and Clayton and beginning to suffer blisters. . . . But he ignored the pain and at the first water station reached for a bottle marked with the radiation hazard symbol. In the bottle was Coca-Cola that he and Kenny Moore had allowed to go flat, so as to avoid stomach cramps from the carbonation. The sugar and caffeine gave him a boot, like a low-budget energy drink. He felt comfortable, his muscles relaxed and his breathing controlled.

*Frank Shorter, winner of the 1972 Munich Olympic Games marathon (Stracher, 2013, pp. 26-27)*

# Does Practice Inform Science, or Does Science Inform Practice?

In the late 1990s, our excitable colleague, Dr. Dave Martin, returned from a professional cycling race with an improbable story. He had documented that professional cycling teams from all around the world were practicing an almost identical strategy. About two-thirds into lengthy races, team soigneurs (handlers) suddenly ditched the sport drink from the team drink bottles and filled them with a defizzed version of a familiar sticky brown liquid. When asked why the cyclists called for this, they answered almost unanimously, "We drink it for the caffeine hit to bring us home with a burst." Huh? Why would you pass over a fluid specifically designed for sport and backed by hundreds of studies showing performance improvements for a lifestyle beverage, albeit heavily marketed and popular?

By our calculations, the amount of caffeine provided by the cola drink was equivalent to 1 to 2 mg/kg and was consumed at the end of the race. This was a far cry from the well-proven caffeine protocols of consuming 6 mg/kg 1 hour prior to an event. It wasn't an entirely new strategy to drink cola during endurance events—Frank Shorter did it on the way to winning the gold medal in the 1972 Olympic Games marathon and it has often been a choice at feed stations in marathons and Ironman races. But at the turn of the century and so systematically, when so much scientific knowledge and assistance was on offer? We just didn't believe it. So, two of the present authors (LB and BD, at that time working together at AIS) put it to the test in two separate investigations. As scientists, we needed to maintain an open mind and see what the data said. However, we assumed that we would be teaching those cyclists a few things.

Our studies were based on a lab protocol lasting about 2.5 hours, with the last 25 minutes undertaken as a time trial. Highly trained cyclists competed on four separate occasions, each undertaken with the nutritional strategies promoted for optimal performance—a prerace meal and sport drink consumed during the race. One trial served as a placebo in which dummy capsules were consumed. The other three trials involved a caffeine dose given in a certain way—the traditional 6 mg/kg taken 1 hour before the start of the trial, 6 mg/kg spread out throughout the race, or the cola strategy, which involved switching from sport drink to cola for the last two bidons of the seven provided throughout the race.

Figure 5.1a shows the results of the time trial from this study and, to our surprise, the ability of the cola drink to improve performance by a margin that was substantial and equivalent to the benefits provided by the larger caffeine doses. Even then we weren't convinced, however. Surely some of this was due to the fact that the cyclists could see they were receiving a cola drink. And of course, the cola drink had a higher carbohydrate content (11% versus 6%), so perhaps the extra muscle fuel was responsible.

We repeated the study again with four new trials. This time, each trial involved switching from sport drink to a cola-flavored beverage for the last two drinks in the trial. These cola beverages looked and tasted identical but had different carbohydrate and caffeine contents—there was a 6% carbohydrate drink to mimic the sport drink and provide our placebo condition, an 11% carbohydrate drink, a 6% carbohydrate drink with the caffeine content of a cola drink, and finally, the real thing

*(continued)*

*(continued)*

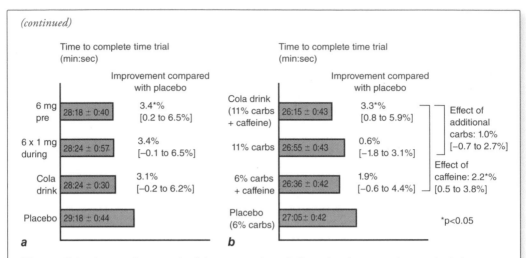

**Figure 5.1** In our first study *(a)*, consuming defizzed cola near the end of the race produced performance improvements comparable to traditional caffeine dosage protocols. Our second study *(b)* showed a similar improvement and demonstrated that the effect owed to the caffeine in the cola rather than the carbohydrate.

with caffeine and 11% carbohydrate. Figure 5.1*b* again tells the story of a consistent 3% improvement in time-trial performance with the real cola drink, and most of the benefit being explained by the small caffeine hit. We learned two unexpected lessons—that practice is sometimes ahead of science, and that small amounts of caffeine are sufficient to enhance performance when taken in a fatigued state.

The story doesn't stop there, though. Even though our results were published in a peer-reviewed journal and open to scrutiny, they still seemed unbelievable to our fellow scientists. So author number 3 (LS) did his own study to add a new dimension. A similar exercise protocol was chosen—120 minutes at ~60% $\dot{V}O_2$max with five hill-climbs at ~85% $\dot{V}O_2$max mixed in, followed by a time trial. In all trials, subjects consumed sport drink throughout the 120-minute cycle. However, at 80 min subjects received one of four treatments in their sport drink: placebo (just the sport drink), CAF1 (100 mg caffeine, ~1.5 mg/kg), CAF2 (200 mg caffeine, ~3 mg/kg), or a random repeat of one of the other three conditions. Subjects completed the time trial in 28:41 ± 0:38 (min:s) in the placebo condition and improved by the statistically significant amount of about 1 minute when they received 100 mg of caffeine (27:36 ± 0:32). They were about another minute faster when they received 200 mg of caffeine (26:36 ± 0:22). Repeated time-trial performances were similar to the original condition, confirming that the results were solid.

Taken together, these results confirm the benefits of very low caffeine doses, especially when introduced as fatigue is becoming apparent, and the maximum benefits occurring with caffeine doses of about 3 mg/kg. But they also speak to the way we cling to our beliefs and need to see things for ourselves before we want to update our ideas. And yes, sometimes, athletes do know best.

consumed during exercise because the fuel source isn't in short supply. However, if only small amounts of carbohydrate are consumed during endurance exercise, the increased availability of this muscle fuel, courtesy of caffeine, may mean better performance outcomes.

Finally, the overwhelming majority of studies on caffeine and endurance performance have provided caffeine in the form of pills or drinks, which require the caffeine to be absorbed from the gut. A more recent study has investigated the effectiveness of caffeinated gum, which allows a more rapid caffeine uptake via direct absorption from the cheek cells. Although the results of this study suggested that the timing of caffeinated gum use might be important in achieving the caffeine benefit, further work is needed before we can be clear about the implications of using this caffeine delivery system.

Here are the key messages from these studies:

- The case for caffeine use in endurance sports seems clear—benefits are likely with small to moderate doses of caffeine. Although doses of 6 mg/kg have been traditional, there is growing evidence that a caffeine dose of 3 mg/kg is enough to get the maximum benefit.

- There are a variety of ways to achieve a beneficial result from caffeine use in endurance sports. These could include taking caffeine before the event, spreading out consumption during the event, or taking it in the late stages of the event just as fatigue is starting to occur. The best option is likely to be specific to the event, the athlete, and the practicalities of caffeine intake.

- Endurance athletes who wish to involve caffeine in their programs should experiment with such protocols to find and fine-tune the practice that will work for them.

- More research should be done to determine useful protocols for a range of sports and to check that the benefits apply to elite athletes in addition to the well-trained performers who have volunteered for studies. Studies on female athletes are also encouraged in order to address their current lack of involvement in caffeine research.

- Caffeine supplementation may interact with other nutritional strategies that are undertaken to promote endurance performance. There is some evidence that the benefits of caffeine supplementation are smaller in situations in which the athlete is well fueled and consumes carbohydrate during the event, but further study on this topic is needed. Another important theme for research is the effect of combining caffeine supplementation with other potentially ergogenic supplements such as creatine, bicarbonate, beetroot juice (nitrate), and beta-alanine.

# Sustained High-Intensity Sports

Sports scientists have also studied the effects of caffeine on events involving higher intensity exercise of shorter duration (see table 5.3 at the end of the chapter). Races in rowing, swimming, middle-distance running, and track endurance cycling typically last 1 to 30 minutes and are conducted at work intensities from around the lactate threshold to above maximal aerobic capacity. Fatigue occurs over the race, and it is possible that caffeine supplementation might help athletes resist this fatigue. Because the duration of the event is so brief, the only practical way to use caffeine is to supplement before the race. In most studies, caffeine doses are taken 1 hour before the race.

The available research supports the potential benefits of caffeine on short, high-intensity sports. Most of the studies have used the traditional caffeine dose (6 mg/kg), but there is some evidence that lower doses (3 mg/kg) may be useful for these events. This is an area that deserves more attention because the competition timetable in many of these events involves multiple races—heats, semis, and finals, for example—and in some cases, the athlete may need to compete more than once in a day. Questions that need answering include the possibility of carryover effects—good or bad—from caffeine use in one race that affect the next one.

So far the research summarized in tables 5.2 and 5.3 has been dominated by the use of conventional statistics to examine and interpret the numbers. However, one study has taken a slightly more athlete-friendly approach to its results. This investigation from sport scientists from Canterbury Christ Church University in England involved a laboratory-based study simulating the 1 km cycling time trial (called the *kilo*) in track cycling. They found that caffeine supplementation improved the kilo performance of well-trained cyclists by an average of 2.4 seconds—a 3.1% improvement in time.

Probability statistics would consider this to be a significant difference; however, the researchers wanted to see what this would mean to the real world of sport. They calculated another statistical concept called *95% confidence limits*—the range in which we could be 95% sure that our results would lie if we repeated the study over and over again with similar groups of cyclists. This calculation produced a performance improvement ranging from 0.7% to 5.6%. The researchers also looked at the results from the men's kilo event at the 2004 Athens Olympic Games to put this into perspective: The difference between the gold- and silver-medal performances was 0.185 seconds or 0.3%, while the difference between first- and tenth-placed competitors was 2.39 seconds or 3.8%. We don't know the variability in the day-to-day performance of these cyclists, but it is likely that the performance benefits of caffeine seen in this study would shine through to make a difference.

Three of the studies within this literature have investigated the interaction of caffeine supplementation with another ergogenic aid, bicarbonate loading, which enhances the athlete's ability to buffer the excess accumulation and flux of hydrogen ions (acidity) out of the muscle as a byproduct of high-intensity exercise. This is a common supplementation strategy practiced by rowers, swimmers, track cyclists, and other athletes who compete in events lasting about 1 to 7 minutes in which changes in muscle acidity contribute to fatigue and performance decline in the late stages of a race. These studies shared the same design in requiring their athletes to undertake four trials—a placebo trial (pretend versions of both supplements), trials in which they received active forms of one of the supplements, and a trial in which both supplements were real. The studies' performance measures and questions were different, and they found different results regarding the interaction of the supplements.

> In the late '80s I gave a presentation to a group of elite Ironman triathletes. Caffeine was one of the hot topics they were keen to hear about. Based on a review of all the evidence, it was unclear whether caffeine was an effective ergogenic aid. This was my conclusion in the presentation. One well-known triathlete asked me if I had ever completed an Ironman triathlon, and my answer was no. He suggested I do one because this would certainly change my conclusion. In his opinion, cola drinks were highly effective in getting him to the finish line in the best time. Almost all of the audience agreed. It took many years until the research caught up with what the athletes had learned from practice. It demonstrates the importance of scientists' listening to the athlete experience.
>
> *Sports dietitian to elite athletes*

The study of rowers found that caffeine supplementation enhanced the performance of a 2,000 m piece undertaken on a rowing ergometer. However, the bicarbonate supplement was associated with gastrointestinal distress that reduced performance and counteracted the gains made when caffeine when used. (Alternatively, you could argue that gains achieved by caffeine supplementation canceled out the performance loss associated with the gut problems caused by bicarbonate loading.)

The other investigation asked swimmers to undertake two 200 m races, 30 min apart, as might occur at a swim meet when competitors race in their main event and a relay, or when they race in the semis of one event and the finals of another on the same program. Caffeine offered a benefit to the performance of the first swim but may have actually impaired the performance of the second one. Sometimes being able to go harder in a first effort in sport has the penalty of making it harder for subsequent efforts. In this study, it looked as if bicarbonate loading was able to rescue the performance of the second swim. Finally, a study of 3 km cycling found that both caffeine and bicarbonate enhanced performance when taken by themselves, but the combination of both did not further improve the outcome. More studies that investigate these real-life challenges and strategies are encouraged.

Here are the key messages to take away from these studies:

- Again, there is good evidence that caffeine intake before an event can enhance the performance of sustained high-intensity sports lasting 1 to 30 min. Higher caffeine doses (6 mg/kg) have received most of the attention to date, and more work is needed to investigate whether low-moderate caffeine doses (up to 3 mg/kg) are equally as effective.

- Many sports that fit under this physiological profile have not been studied in relation to the potential benefits of caffeine. As usual, work on elite performers is lacking and female athletes are also underrepresented.

- The logistics of competition in these events raises some issues. How should an athlete who has several races in a day or over several days of competition tackle a repeated caffeine dose? Issues that need to be considered include the duration of the effect of caffeine and whether a caffeine dose needs to be repeated or topped up over a day or session of competition. The issue of sleep quality after caffeine use and the effect on next day's performance also needs to be considered.

- Interaction with other supplements and nutrition strategies needs to be studied.

- The effect of too much caffeine on overarousal and interference with technique should be considered in sports that involve a high degree of skill (e.g., swimming, rowing).

- Plans for caffeine use need to be developed on an individual basis for athletes.

## Stop-and-Go Sports

Research on team and racket sports faces some extra challenges. It's just about impossible to do a fully controlled crossover field study, where players perform with one condition in one match and then the opposite intervention on the next occasion. It's not just about changes in the weather, the encouragement of the crowd, or other external factors that affect the outcomes of a sport such as a marathon. Unlike a marathon, which is always 42.195 km, each match is literally a new ball game! You can't play it twice or three times. Researchers have tried to get around this by developing batteries of tests that mimic the key characteristics of a team or racket sport. Sometimes it is just about the stop–start running patterns, with researchers testing out speed, the development of fatigue over repeated sprints, and agility. Other times, tests of skill and concentration are added. New methodologies such as global positioning satellite (GPS) monitoring now provide options to allow some dimensions of real games to be measured – such as time and distance spent running at different speeds. Of course, the limit in measuring running patterns or skill execution is the leap of faith that these elements underpin the activities that decide the outcome of a match—goals scored or winning shots played.

There are now quite a few studies on the effect of caffeine supplementation on elements or simulations of team and racket sports (table 5.4 at the end of the chapter). Most of these have used the traditional caffeine protocol—6 mg/kg taken 1 hour before the start of play, although more recent studies have used the new caffeine benchmark dose of 3 mg/kg. This is a pity, because most team and racket sports offer opportunities for a variety of ways to take caffeine for a match—there are usually many breaks in play in which drinks and other products can be consumed. We would like to see more studies that use the lower caffeine dose that spreads it out over the event, or that wait until the second half or later stages of a match when the player is becoming fatigued.

We expect that a range of protocols might work for different individuals within team and racket sports. For example, some players would benefit from finding the lowest effective caffeine dose for games played at night so that the disturbance to postmatch sleep is minimized. Other players might be better off avoiding the mixture of a buzz from pre-event caffeine with the adrenalin rush associated with running out onto the ground or court and engaging with the crowd and opponents. This would allow them to quickly settle into the desirable level of concentration and technique rather than being overstimulated. It would also offer the addition of caffeine to their match nutrition strategies to stave off fatigue at the business end of the game.

One investigation of football (soccer), conducted by Spanish researcher, Juan Del Coso and summarized in table 5.4 provides information that is symbolic of the newer studies of caffeine and stop-and-go sports. The study design ticks a number of boxes—it involved reasonably good and experienced subjects (semiprofessional players), controlled a lot of factors that might influence performance, and combined some controllable tests (measures

> I drink Red Bull to help my training and concentration, and being fit means you'll give your all to win for England.
>
> *Kevin Pietersen, cricket player and former captain of the English cricket team (Newman, 2009)*

of a player's ability to jump to head the ball and a repeated sprint protocol) as well as observations of movement patterns in some real-life games. Caffeine was provided via a well-known energy drink; a sugar-free form was chosen to remove the effect of carbohydrate on performance. The caffeine dose was moderate (3 mg/kg), provided by about 630 ml of the energy drink and consumed 1 hour before the start of the tests. Two games were played, each with half of the players on each side receiving caffeine and the other half getting a placebo noncaffeinated version of the drink, and the test battery was undertaken before the start of each game.

The results from the study showed clear evidence of better performance when caffeine was present in the pregame drink—players performed better in the battery of tests as well as achieving better running outcomes in the games. Specifically, they ran farther in the games, ran greater distances at higher intensities, and walked less. Analysis of the outcomes for individual players showed that 17 of the 19 who completed the study were responders to caffeine, improving on at least two of the three measures. The other two did not appear to benefit overall. Postgame urine tests revealed a mean urinary caffeine concentration of 4.1 µg/ml—well below the old antidoping threshold of 12 µg/ml.

Here are the key messages of these studies:

- Benefits from caffeine supplementation in team and racket sports seem to be most likely when the match would otherwise reduce performance across play. These benefits might be seen in terms of the amount and speed of running that is done or the execution of skills and concentration.

- Studies should try to measure the effects of caffeine on the match-winning aspects of these sports (e.g., number of goals scored or conceded, winning shots, unforced errors). Field studies are presently rare.

- Caffeine studies should focus on protocols that use low-moderate doses and protocols in which the caffeine is spread out during the match. Fluid and fuel levels in these sports may also limit performance, so competition strategies should include or measure the independent effects of hydration, carbohydrate intake, and the use of other evidence-based supplements (e.g., bicarbonate, beta-alanine, beetroot juice).

- Negative effects on sleep and overarousal are possible and should be considered.

- Studies need to include high-caliber athletes and female athletes, who are underrepresented in research projects.

- Plans for caffeine use need to be developed on an individual basis, even in team sports.

# Placebo Effects and Caffeine

One of the key factors in well-conducted studies is a placebo control, which takes into account the well-known effect that when people are given something special or treated in a special way, they change their behaviors, efforts, and abilities. We all know of situations in which people try a new supplement or intervention and swear that it has changed their life, even when there is no sound reason for a change to occur. Even being monitored or having performance measured in a study or in a laboratory can make people pull out a best performance because they respond to the special attention. These outcomes are examples of the placebo effect, which is often described as the power of positive thinking. In other words, it is a change that occurs because of the belief of the person who receives attention.

The placebo effect should not be disparaged or considered imaginary. Studies show that belief can cause real changes in the brain and body, producing substantial changes in health, performance, or other objective measures. Understanding and measuring the size of effects caused by belief or placebo is a science emerging in its own importance. In the meantime, good sports scientists look for strategies that can enhance performance by adding a placebo-inspired improvement on top of a physiological change. This way an athlete gets the best of both worlds or double the benefits of any treatment.

In the research setting, scientists know that they must include strategies within their studies to account for any effects that are achieved by belief rather than by the intervention alone. This means that research projects can't simply provide subjects with a supplement (or other intervention), measure performance before and after, and expect to isolate the true effect of the supplement. After all, at least some of the change that occurs after trialing the supplement occurs because subjects expect a change to occur or are on their best behavior because they are being observed.

To control for this, the project should involve a trial or group receiving a dummy treatment, whereby the only effect that can occur is because of belief. The difference in effect between the trials involving the real supplement and the placebo supplement is due to the supplement itself. Ideally, the supplement and the placebo are identical in look, taste, texture, and whatever other characteristics are superficially identifiable. The best projects quiz subjects after their trials to see if they can guess which treatment they took. Hopefully, the results suggest a pure guess so that the identity of the placebo treatment was not broken. The studies of caffeine and performance that have been included in our review have all included placebo treatments in their design. Many of them also checked to see how well they did in disguising the placebo treatment so that subjects believed they were receiving the real thing.

That's not the end of the story, though, when it comes to placebos and caffeine. Some intriguing studies have been conducted by Dr. Chris Beedie and colleagues at Canterbury Christ Church University, showing that people have such strong

*(continued)*

*(continued)*

perceptions about caffeine that they can produce measurable effects on performance. In one study, cyclists undertook a baseline trial followed by three time trials in which they were told they would be receiving no caffeine in one trial, a moderate dose in another (4.5 mg/kg), and a large dose in the third (9 mg/kg). The cyclists didn't know which order the trials would be in, but most importantly, they didn't know that all of the treatments provided in each trial were placebos—no caffeine was consumed at all! Before they received feedback, subjects nominated which of their trials corresponded to the caffeine dose received. Remarkably, when compared with the baseline time trial, they produced 1.4% less power in the effort in which they believed they had not received any caffeine, 1.3% more power when they believed they had received the moderate caffeine dose, and 3% more power when they thought they had received the large dose of caffeine. Not only could they make the imagined caffeine work when they believed they had taken it, but they could also make it work better at higher doses!

What happens, though, when people receive caffeine without knowing it? Dr. Beedie's group had cyclists complete four 40 km time trials under varying conditions. On two occasions, they received a caffeine dose—once after being told they were being given caffeine, and once after being told they were not. Similarly, on another two occasions, they received a placebo treatment with instructions that they were either getting caffeine or not getting it. The caffeine treatment improved mean power by 3.5%, and just being told they were receiving caffeine provided a 0.7% boost. However, the effect of caffeine was reduced when subjects were told they weren't getting it and the belief in caffeine produced a better effect when no caffeine was consumed. There was a possible harmful effect of not receiving caffeine and being told of this—mean power was decreased by 1.9%. Thus it seemed that a negative expectation was more powerful than a positive expectation. The bottom line is that the brain is a powerful organ in directing sports performance, and we invest heavily in our beliefs about what caffeine can do for us.

## Strength and Power Events

Few studies have examined the effect of caffeine supplementation on explosive power or strength in trained populations (see table 5.5 at the end of the chapter for a summary of studies involving single maximal efforts or sprints shorter than 20 seconds that relate to sport). Furthermore, the available studies rely on measuring maximal strength for single effort in gym settings rather than applying it to a sport—for example, a throw, lift, jump, or sprint event in track cycling or athletics. The evidence for a benefit from caffeine, at least when 6 mg/kg doses are taken by resistance-trained people, is unclear and may be limited to upper-body movements. The only investigation of well-trained athletes in a field setting using small doses of caffeine from a rapidly absorbed source (gum) reported apparent benefits to shot-put performance. Clearly, more studies are needed in this area to see if caffeine can make an athlete stronger, higher, or faster in the purest sense of sport.

Although we haven't specifically reviewed the studies in this area, there is some evidence that caffeine supplementation enhances muscular endurance—athletes might do more reps to failure in the gym or a better workout of repeated sprints at the track or velodrome. This might explain the popularity of consuming preworkout supplements or coffee before a gym or track workout. Apart from undertaking more sport-specific studies to determine whether caffeine assists the performance of such workouts, it would be good to measure the accumulated effect of better workouts on the performance of lifts, sprints, or throws on competition day. The effect of repeated efforts on performance on competition day—for example, each of the jumps or throws in a round of competition or the individual events in a decathlon or heptathlon—is also of interest.

Here are the key messages from these studies:

- This type of sporting activity seems least likely to benefit from caffeine supplementation, although more studies of sport-specific situations and well-trained participants are encouraged.
- The situations in which caffeine supplementation might be most likely to benefit the performance of strength and power sports might relate to strength and power endurance—for example, multiple repetitions of lifts during training or repeated throws, jumps, or lifts in competition.
- More research is encouraged since the effects of caffeine on strength and power are relatively less explored.

## Skill Sports

Finally, there is potential for caffeine to enhance the performance of sports that rely heavily on skill, such as golf, shooting, and archery. Even when these sports do not involve fatiguing exercise per se, their events are often conducted over lengthy periods in harsh conditions during which competitors are likely to feel mentally and physically fatigued. The available studies involving skill-focused sports (see table 5.6 at the end of the chapter) do not show clear evidence of benefits from caffeine supplementation, but they also show that the scenario has not been addressed well. Note that inappropriately large intakes of caffeine cause symptoms of jitters and anxiety in many people, which would be expected to impair fine motor control and concentration. Therefore, researchers who take up the call to monitor skill sports and caffeine intake should concentrate on protocols involving small-moderate caffeine servings.

Here are the key messages regarding skill sports:

- This type of sport has received the least amount of attention with regard to caffeine and should be explored.
- Protocols of caffeine use should focus on small-moderate doses to reduce any side effects of caffeine on fine motor control.

# Caffeine and the Effectiveness of Training

Competition performance is the result of a series of enhancements that have been made possible through the training process. Athletes train to produce improvements in all the various aspects of the physiology, biomechanics, psychology, and nutrition that underpin the final outcome of their event. In effect, training is a periodized program of progressive overload and event simulation that focuses on producing the best outcome on certain days. Each of the workouts or practice events that contribute to this peak is likely to involve an exercise activity that fits into one of the categories that were reviewed previously in this chapter. As we have seen, caffeine intake may enhance the performance of that activity, allowing the athlete to finish it sooner, with less fatigue, with better form, or with greater work in the given time. Therefore, it makes sense to think that caffeine could become part of the training formula. Certainly, there are caffeine products marketed specifically for this purpose, such as preworkout supplements. (Note, however, that we have expressed some concerns about many of these products due to their unclear labeling and the presence of other stimulants, including substances that are banned under the WADA code.)

Unfortunately, although it is likely that caffeine supplementation can enhance the outcome of a single training session, no studies have systematically studied the influence of the chronic use of caffeine on the effectiveness of a training block and its ultimate transfer into competition performance. It is likely that there are potential advantages and disadvantages of using caffeine as an ergogenic aid for each training session. In chapter 10, we will work through the pros and the cons of using caffeine to promote performance in training sessions, with particular interest in timing your existing caffeine intake or your training sessions so that they are a good match for each other. See the sidebar on train-low tactics (Can Caffeine Rescue Train-Low Tactics?) for an example of sessions that might benefit from this approach.

## Can Caffeine Rescue Train-Low Tactics?

A new concept in sport nutrition is the practice of training low. This isn't in reference to altitude or mood but rather the deliberate decision to undertake some training sessions with low muscle glycogen stores or the absence of carbohydrate-fueling strategies. Clearly this is counter to the principles of competition nutrition, where being well fueled with carbohydrate is important for top performance of the muscles and the mind. However, recent research has shown that the muscle has a different response to exercise undertaken with low carbohydrate reserves. The muscle cell experiences an amplified stimulus, as shown by a larger production of signaling chemicals and an increased synthesis of the proteins that make it more suited to exercise. Studies show that repeating this strategy produces muscle with more of the enzyme machinery that promotes the capacity for exercise.

This strategy might be put into practice by doing two training sessions close together so that the second one is done without the ability to refuel from the first or training first thing in the morning after an overnight fast and without any carbohydrate intake. It all sounds promising, except that no study of this train-low strategy in already trained people has shown that it leads to a better performance outcome than conventional training does. One of the possible reasons is that training low is associated with a lower intensity of training because the athlete feels fatigued. Perhaps the lack of high-intensity work cancels out the other benefits.

A new thought is to try to rescue the impaired training sessions with strategies to help fatigued athletes train harder. Caffeine, anyone? Stephen Lane, a doctoral student at the Royal Melbourne Institute of Technology (RMIT University) in Melbourne, has put this to the test, measuring the self-chosen training intensity when cyclists are required to do an interval training session under varying conditions—with high muscle glycogen or with low muscle glycogen due to differences in the time for refueling after a previous glycogen-depleting workout. The interval session is one commonly undertaken by endurance athletes and involves eight intervals undertaken as hard as possible, with a one-minute recovery between each. The results showed a clear hierarchy of effort. When the athletes had to train low with depleted glycogen levels, they were unable to work as hard as when they were well fueled as shown by drop of nearly 9% in average power output. Adding caffeine to the low glycogen partially rescued the session by increasing training intensity by 3.5%. Meanwhile, adding caffeine to the fully fuelled training achieved the best outcome of all, with the average power output increasing by an extra 2.8% while giving the same perception of effort (see figure 5.2). Whether the chronic combination of caffeine and with-low-fuel workouts leads to a better training outcome deserves to be tested.

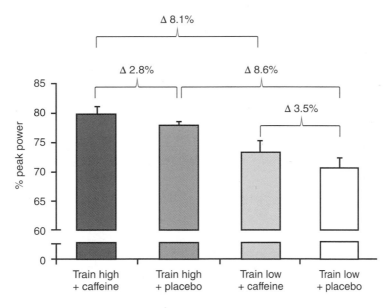

**Figure 5.2** Studies showing the effect of caffeine supplementation on power outputs in high-intensity interval sessions undertaken while well fueled or using a train-low protocol that may enhance the training response. The values show the average power selected for the intervals as a percentage of the athlete's peak power output. Low-glycogen training significantly impairs high-intensity training, while taking caffeine before the session rescues this effect to small but worthwhile extent. Even when the athlete is well-fuelled, caffeine still increases the self-chosen exercise intensity for the session.

# The Bottom Line

There are lots of studies related to caffeine and exercise, but only a subset of these provides a useful examination of caffeine and sports performance. There is a need for many new studies to better explore the effects of caffeine on the outcomes of specific sports, and these investigations should include features that make their results easy to translate into the real world. Differences in caffeine protocols need to be explored, including the timing and amount of the dose and the source of caffeine. Factors that need to be included in studies include the effect of adding other nutritional strategies such as consuming carbohydrate before and during the event and using other proven ergogenic aids.

In the meantime, there is evidence that caffeine supplementation can improve performance or the outcomes of a range of sporting events, particularly those involving a prolonged duration of sustained or intermittent efforts. Furthermore, it appears that these benefits are achieved, or even maximized, from small to moderate doses of caffeine (up to 3 mg/kg), and in longer events, a range of caffeine protocols might be equally effective. Of course, results differ according to the individual athlete. But before this information can be put into action, we need to consider other effects that caffeine might have on the implementation of a training or competition plan.

**Table 5.1** Spot the Difference! Traditional Laboratory-Based Research Versus Research Focused on Elite Sports Performance

| Features of traditional studies | Features of elite and serious sport | Translating from the study to sport |
|---|---|---|
| Subjects are usually recruited from available populations such as students in the researcher's university or local groups of recreational or moderately trained subjects. | Athletes are highly trained in their sport and event.<br>• They are reliable in repeating a given performance task.<br>• They are specifically adapted to their sport through natural selection and the conditioning effects of training. | Have faith that you can best translate the results of a study to a population that is similar to the one in the study.<br><br>Be careful about expecting that results seen in one group can apply to another—for example, that elite athletes will respond exactly the same way as recreational subjects or that well-trained subjects are the same as junior competitors. |
| Exercise protocols typically measure endurance or exercise capacity (the ability to sustain a given exercise task for as long as possible). The task is terminated when the subject is fatigued and unable to continue at the prescribed intensity or speed. | Sports performance typically includes the following:<br>• Completing a distance in the fastest possible time. Pace judgment is important.<br>• Executing a single task as well as possible.<br>• Executing skills and making complex decisions while undertaking exercise.<br>Training situations may better represent the execution of exercise to fatigue. | Pay most attention to studies that best mimic a real-life event, but even then remember that not all aspects of a sport decide the outcome of the event. For example, it might be useful for a team-sport player to be able to run faster in the last minutes of a match, but this needs to translate into more goals scored to be truly valuable. |

| Features of traditional studies | Features of elite and serious sport | Translating from the study to sport |
| --- | --- | --- |
| Exercise is often undertaken with baseline metabolic conditions—subjects fast overnight and consume only water during exercise. Subjects may also be required to avoid all other confounding variables, such as the use of other supplements. | Athletes undertake other nutrition strategies that provide additional support for performance:<br>• Following a carbohydrate-rich pre-event meal<br>• Consuming carbohydrate during prolonged events<br>• Using other scientifically supported ergogenic aids (e.g., bicarbonate, creatine, beta-alanine, beetroot juice) | Pay most attention to studies that best mimic the real-life practices of athletes, including their usual strategies of fueling up before and during an event.<br>Consider the interaction of caffeine use with other nutritional strategies (e.g., the use of other supplements). Ideally, studies will systematically tackle the addition and interaction of various layers of nutrition practice, but until these are done, you may have to factor in the likely outcomes yourself. |
| Differences in performance between the control treatment and the active treatment are assessed using probability statistics; the probability that a difference between the results of the trials could have happened by chance must be less than an arbitrary level (usually a 5% probability) to be considered significant. | The margins between winning and losing, or between the podium athletes and the rest of the field, can often be measured in hundredths of seconds and millimeters. | Pay most attention to studies that use special analyses that take into account the size of the change in performance caused by caffeine in relation to real-life performances. |
| Statistical analyses typically look at a group outcome—the typical response. | In real life, people respond differently to various practices. Sporting competitions give their rewards and recognition to the best few, not the typical performer. | Consider the typical results seen in the study, but be prepared that you might respond differently.<br>Pay attention to studies with larger numbers of subjects in which attention can be paid to the levels of response. Sometimes researchers are able to tease out factors that cause people to fall into categories of nonresponders, responders, and even super-responders. |
| Protocols are shaped according to the concerns of the ethics committee overseeing the project. | Sports are conducted within the regulations of their governing bodies, including antidoping codes and rules that govern playing times and access to nutrition. | Pay most attention to studies that test the practices that are allowable within real-life sport. |
| Subjects often undertake their trials individually. Biological samples—blood, sweat, muscle, breath—may be collected at various time points, including during the exercise task. Subjects may also be required to describe their perceptions of effort, discomfort, or fatigue. These activities may interfere with the subject's ability to exercise at optimal intensity. | Athletes focus on their performance, usually without external interference. They may be distracted or motivated by the performance of other athletes. | Although it is nice to know about the other information collected in studies (for example, what happened to blood markers or muscle fuel use), pay special attention to studies that focus just on performance, especially those that study real-life competition. |

*Note:* For a continually updated version of tables 5.2-5.6, see AIS Sports Supplement Program resources at www.ausport.gov.au/ais/nutrition.

**Table 5.2**  Does Caffeine Enhance the Performance of Endurance Sports Lasting Longer Than 60 Minutes?

| Study | Subjects[a] | Caffeine intake (amount and timing of intake in relation to the event) | Measurement of sports performance | Was it enhanced? | Technical comments |
|-------|----------|-------------------------------------------------------------------------|-----------------------------------|------------------|--------------------|
| | | | CYCLING | | |
| Hodgson et al. 2013 | Well-trained cyclists/triathletes (8 M) | Dose: 5 mg/kg Timing: 60 min pre-event 2 caffeine trials: caffeine powder and instant coffee 2 non-caffeine trials: placebo and decaffeinated coffee | 30 min cycling at 55% $\dot{V}O_2$max + TT lasting ~ 45 min | Yes | Both caffeine trials enhanced performance of the TT equally: Caffeine trial was 4.9% faster [95% confidence interval = 2.3–6.8%] and 4.5% [2.3–6.2%] than placebo and decaf (p < 0.05 for both). Equally, coffee significantly improved TT performance by 4.7% [2.3–6.7%] and 4.3% [2.5–7.1%] compared to placebo and decaf. There were no differences between finishing times for caffeine and coffee. |
| Ryan et al. 2013 | Well-trained cyclists (8 M) | Dose: 300 mg (~3 mg/kg) Timing: 120 min, 60 min, and 5 min pre-event Caffeine provided in caffeinated chewing gum, allowing rapid mouth absorption of caffeine. | 15 min cycling at 75% $\dot{V}O_2$max + 7 kJ/kg TT *Information on intake during exercise protocol not provided* | Yes for 5 min No for 60 min No for 120 min | Plasma caffeine concentrations had plateaued at commencement of exercise in 60 and 120 min trials, whereas they continued to rise during cycling when the caffeine was consumed 5 min before starting. Performance was improved in the 5 min trial (38.7 ± 1.2 min, $p = .027$) vs. placebo (40.7 ± 1.2 min) but unchanged in the 60 min (41.8 ± 2.6 min) and 120 min trials (42.6 ± 2.2 min). |
| Skinner et al. 2013 | Well-trained cyclists, triathletes (14 M) | Dose: 6 mg/kg Timing: 60 min pre-event or pre-event such that individual peak plasma caffeine levels coincided with beginning of event (~120 min for 12 subjects and 150 min for 2 subjects) | 40 km TT *Water consumed during exercise protocol* | Yes for 60 min No for peak caffeine | Compared with the placebo trial, taking caffeine 60 min before the time trial enhanced performance by 70.5 s or 2% ($p = .002$). The trial in which the same amount of caffeine was taken to coincide the start of the TT with peak blood caffeine measures showed only a small and nonsignificant performance enhancement (1.1%; $p = .240$). The reasons for this are unclear. |

| Study | Subjects[a] | Caffeine intake (amount and timing of intake in relation to the event) | Measurement of sports performance | Was it enhanced? | Technical comments |
|---|---|---|---|---|---|
| Lassiter et al. 2013 | Trained cyclists (8 M, 7 F) | Dose: 160 mg<br>Timing: 40 min pre-event<br>Caffeine consumed as energy drink with carbohydrate and taurine; placebo = non-caffeinated non-caloric beverage | 35 km TT on ergometer + psychomotor tests (pre-caffeine, post-caffeine and post-TT)<br>• decision making<br>• precision<br>• reaction time<br>• movement time | Yes<br><br><br><br><br>No<br>No<br>Yes<br>Yes | Every subject improved their performance of the 35 km TT with the mean improvement being 3% (2.0±1.3 min; $p < .05$). Improvements were seen both in subjects who came in to trial with high baseline levels of blood caffeine and those who had low baseline concentrations. Enhancement of some cognitive/psychomotor tests was also seen. Effects cannot be totally attributed to caffeine, since the energy drink also contained carbohydrate and other ingredients (e.g., taurine) |
| Acker-Hewitt et al. 2012 | Well-trained cyclists (10 M) | Dose: 6 mg/kg<br>Timing: 60 min pre-event<br>4 trials: caffeine, caffeine + carbohydrate, carbohydrate, and placebo | 15 min cycling at 60% Wmax + 20 km TT<br><br>*Carbohydrate consumed during exercise protocol in some trials* | Yes but only when combined with carbohydrate | The combination of carbohydrate and caffeine enhanced performance of the 20 km TT with a 5% increase in power output and 3.4% reduction in time (42.7 ± 3.9 min, $p < .05$) vs. placebo (44.2 ± 4.5 min). Performance was unchanged with caffeine alone (43.6 ± 4.9 min) and carbohydrate alone (43.8 ± 4.1 min). |
| Desbrow et al. 2012 | Well-trained cyclists (16 M) | Dose: 3 or 6 mg/kg<br>Timing: 90 min pre-event | TT of set work ~65 min<br><br>*Carbohydrate consumed during exercise protocol* | Yes at both doses | 3 mg/kg caffeine enhanced performance by 5.2% and 6 mg/kg by 2.9%. Difference in performance between the caffeine trials was not significant ($p = .24$). |
| Roelands et al. 2011 | Trained cyclists (13 M) | Dose: 6 mg/kg<br>Timing: 60 min pre-event<br>Hot environment: 30 °C (86 °F) | 60 min cycling at 55% Wmax + TT lasting ~30 min<br><br>*Water consumed during exercise protocol* | No | Caffeine ingestion was associated with an increase in rectal temperature. Large performance variability among subjects was noted. |
| Ganio et al. 2011 | Trained cyclists (11 M) | Dose: 6 mg/kg<br>Timing: 3 mg taken 60 min pre-event + 3 mg at 45 min of exercise<br>Cool environment: 12 °C (54 °F)<br>Hot environment: 33 °C (91 °F) | 90 min cycling at 55% Wmax + 15 min TT<br><br>*Water consumed during exercise protocol* | Yes at both temperatures | Performance was substantially reduced in hot (191 ± 35 kJ) compared with cool conditions (237 ± 37 kJ, $p < .05$). However, caffeine ingestion was associated with better performance in each condition compared with the respective placebo trial. This effect was smaller than the effect of temperature (mean = 219 ± 44 kJ for caffeine and 209 ± 42 placebo, $p < .05$). |

*(continued)*

**Table 5.2** *(continued)*

| Study | Subjects[a] | Caffeine intake (amount and timing of intake in relation to the event) | Measurement of sports performance | Was it enhanced? | Technical comments |
|---|---|---|---|---|---|
| CYCLING *(continued)* | | | | | |
| Irwin et al. 2011 | Trained cyclists (11 M) | Dose: 3 mg/kg Timing: 90 min pre-event 4 trials: placebo-controlled caffeine withdrawal or no withdrawal with caffeine vs. placebo during cycling | TT ~60 min *Carbohydrate consumed during exercise protocol* | Yes | Moderate intakes of caffeine were associated with enhanced TT performance irrespective of whether a 4 d caffeine withdrawal was imposed. Improvement was 3% in the caffeine withdrawal trials (~1:49 min, $p = .02$) and 3.6% with the nonwithdrawal trials (~2:07 min, $p < .002$). Subjects were blinded to the withdrawal; self-reported symptoms were mild and inconsistently seen. |
| Desbrow et al. 2009 | Trained cyclists (9 M) | Dose: 3 mg/kg or 1.5 mg/kg Timing: 1 h pre-event | 120 min cycling at 70% $\dot{V}O_2$max + 7 kJ/kg TT (~30 min) *Carbohydrate consumed during exercise protocol* | No | Small trend to enhanced performance with 3 mg/kg dose (29 min: 51 s ± 3:38; 30:25 ± 3:10 and 30:42 ± 3:41 for 0, 1.5, and 3 mg/kg doses). No difference in muscle utilization of carbohydrate drink consumed during trial as seen in other studies; it was suggested that effect on carbohydrate utilization only occurs if carbohydrate intake is below optimal amounts. |
| Ivy et al. 2009 | Trained cyclists (6 M, 6 F) | Dose: 160 mg Timing: 40 min pre-event Caffeine provided as energy drink with taurine and other ingredients. | TT ~60 min *Carbohydrate provided in pre-event drink but water consumed during TT* | Yes | Performance was improved with pre-event caffeine (3,690 s vs. 3,874 s, $p < .01$). No differences in RPE were seen. |
| Cureton et al. 2007 | Well-trained cyclists (16 M) | Dose: 5.3 mg/kg Timing: 1.2 mg/kg pre-event + 0.6 mg/kg every 15 min during cycling | 120 min cycling at 60 and 75% $\dot{V}O_2$max + 15 min TT *Carbohydrate consumed during exercise protocol* | Yes | Exercise intensity during the 15 min time trial was higher with caffeine + carbohydrate (90% $\dot{V}O_2$max ± 11%) vs. carbohydrate alone (79% $\dot{V}O_2$max ± 14 %). |
| Conway, Orr, and Stannard 2003 | Trained cyclists and triathletes (9 M) | Dose and timing: • 6 mg/kg 60 min pre-event • 3 mg/kg pre-event + 3 mg/kg at 45 min during event | 90 min cycling at 68% $\dot{V}O_2$max + TT (~30 min) | Perhaps | There was a trend to better TT performance with caffeine trials (24.2 and 23.4 min) vs. placebo (28.3 min), $p = .08$. |

| Study | Subjects[a] | Caffeine intake (amount and timing of intake in relation to the event) | Measurement of sports performance | Was it enhanced? | Technical comments |
|---|---|---|---|---|---|
| Hunter et al. 2002 | Highly trained cyclists (8 M) | Dose: 6 mg/kg Timing: 60 min pre-event + 0.33 mg/kg every 15 min | 100 km cycling TT including 5 × 1 km and 4 × 4 km efforts<br><br>*Carbohydrate consumed during exercise protocol* | No | Differences between trials in terms of total 100 km time or time to complete 1 km and 4 km high-intensity efforts were minimal. |
| Cox et al. 2002 | Well-trained cyclists and triathletes (12 M) | Dose and timing:<br>• 6 mg/kg 60 min pre-event<br>• 6 × 1 mg every 20 min during exercise<br>• 10 ml/kg Coca-Cola in last 50 min (~1-1.5 mg/kg caffeine) | 120 min cycling at 70% $\dot{V}O_2$max + 7 kJ/kg TT (~30 min)<br><br>*Carbohydrate consumed during exercise protocol* | Yes at all doses | Large dose caffeine (6 mg/kg) improved TT performance by 3% over placebo trial TT regardless of timing of intake. Coca-Cola consumed late in exercise (~1 mg/kg caffeine) produced equal improvement. Urinary caffeine levels were ~4-5 µg/ml for large dose caffeine and <1 µ/ml for cola. |
| Cox et al. 2002 | Well-trained cyclists and triathletes (8 M) | Sport drink replaced during last 70 min by 15 ml/kg of a cola-flavored drink:<br>• 6% carbohydrate<br>• 11% carbohydrate<br>• 6% carbohydrate + 13 mg/100 ml caffeine<br>• 11% carbohydrate + 13 mg/100 ml caffeine (Coca-Cola)<br>Caffeine dose ~1.5 mg/kg | 2 h cycling at 70% $\dot{V}O_2$max + 7 kJ/kg TT (~30 min)<br><br>*Carbohydrate consumed during exercise protocol* | Yes | Coca-Cola consumed late in exercise produced 3% performance benefit in TT compared with cola-flavored placebo drink. Benefits were explained by caffeine content (~2%) and increased carbohydrate intake (~1%). |
| Jacobson et al. 2001 | Trained cyclists (8 M) | Dose: 6 mg/kg Timing: 60 min pre-event 4 trials: caffeine, carbohydrate, caffeine + carbohydrate, placebo | 120 min cycling at 70% $\dot{V}O_2$max + 7 kJ/kg TT (~30 min)<br><br>*Carbohydrate consumed during some exercise protocols* | No | TT performance was similar in caffeine + carbohydrate trial (29.12 min) and carbohydrate trial (30.12 min), but both trials were better than placebo. |
| Ivy et al. 1979 | Trained cyclists (7M, 2F) | Dose: 500 mg Timing: 250 mg at 60 min pre-event + 250 mg spread into 7 doses during exercise | 120 min isokinetic cycling at 80 rpm | Yes | 7% increase in total work with caffeine trial compared with placebo. Perception of effort was the same in each trial despite increased work with caffeine. |
| Kovacs, Stegen, and Brouns 1998 | Well-trained cyclists (15 M) | Dose:<br>• 2.1 mg/kg<br>• 3.2 mg/kg<br>• 4.5 mg/kg<br>Timing: spread between 75 min pre-event + 20 and 40 min of TT | Cycling TT (~1 h)<br><br>*Carbohydrate consumed during exercise protocols* | Yes at all doses | Addition of caffeine to sport drinks improved TT performance. The benefits with 3.2 and 4.5 mg/kg caffeine were equal and were greater than with 2.1 mg/kg. Urinary caffeine levels reflected total dose, but all were below 12 µg/ml. |

*(continued)*

**Table 5.2** *(continued)*

| Study | Subjects[a] | Caffeine intake (amount and timing of intake in relation to the event) | Measurement of sports performance | Was it enhanced? | Technical comments |
|---|---|---|---|---|---|
| CROSS-COUNTRY SKIING | | | | | |
| Berglund and Hemmingsson 1982 | Well-trained cross-country skiers (14 M) | Dose: 6 mg/kg Timing: pre-event | 21 km cross-country ski race Field study <br> • Low altitude <br> • High altitude | Perhaps Yes | Individual race times were expressed as % of mean race time to account for differences in weather between trials. At low altitude, there was a trend to better performance with caffeine. At halfway point, time was decreased by 0.9% of mean race time (~33 s) compared with placebo ($p < .05$). At full distance, decrease was 1.7% of the mean time (~59 s) ($p < .1$). At high altitudes, the race time was significantly faster with caffeine than with placebo (**$p < .001$**) both after one lap (2.2% or ~101 s) and two laps (3.2% or ~152 s). |
| DISTANCE RUNNING | | | | | |
| Cohen et al. 1996 | Trained runners (5 M, 2 F) | Dose: <br> • 5 mg/kg <br> • 9 mg/kg <br> Timing: pre-event | Half-marathon = 21 km Field study | No | No effects on RPE or performance at either dose compared with placebo. |
| Van Nieuwenhoven, Brouns, and Kovacs 2005 | Trained to well-trained runners (90 M, 8 F) | Dose: ~1.3 mg/kg Timing: divided between prerace + 4.5, 9, and 13.5 km of race 3 trials: caffeine + carbohydrate, carbohydrate, water | 18 km road-running race field study *Carbohydrate consumed during race in some trials* | No | No differences in performance of whole group between caffeinated sport drink (78:03 ± 8:42 [min:s]), sport drink (78:23 ± 8:47), or water (78:03 ± 8:30) or for 10 fastest runners (63:41 and 63:54, vs. 63:50 for caffeine sport drink, sport drink, and water, respectively). |

[a] Unless otherwise stated, all studies used a crossover design in which subjects acted as their own controls, undertaking both the caffeine and placebo trial; TT = time trial. M = males, F = females. Wmax = Maximal work output (Watts)

**Table 5.3** Does Caffeine Improve the Performance of Sustained High-Intensity Sports Lasting 1 to 30 Minutes?

| Study | Subjects[a] | Caffeine intake | Measurement of sports performance | Was it enhanced? | Technical comments |
|---|---|---|---|---|---|
| MIDDLE DISTANCE AND DISTANCE RUNNING | | | | | |
| O'Rourke, O'Brien, Knez, and Paton 2008 | Well-trained club runners (15 M) and recreational runners (15 M) | Dose: 5 mg/kg Timing: 60 min pre-event | 5K race on track | Yes for well-trained Probably for recreational runners | Caffeine enhanced performance of 5K in well-trained runners by 1.0% (90% CI = 0.4%-1.6%; 1298 ± 84 s vs. 1286 ± 86 s for placebo and caffeine trials, respectively). A similar improvement of 1.1% (90% CI = 0.2%-2%; 1058 ± 68 s vs. 1047 ± 69 s) was seen in recreational runners. Since the reliability of performance in recreational runners was lower (test–retest error = 1.4%), the effect of caffeine may not be so clearly seen. |
| Bridge and Jones 2006 | Distance runners (8 M) | Dose: 3 mg/kg Timing: 60 min pre-event | 8 km race on track | Yes | Compared with a control and placebo trial, caffeine supplementation resulted in a 23.8 s or 1.2% improvement in run time ($p < .05$) with individual results ranging from 10 to 61 s improvement. |
| Wiles, Bird, Hopkins, and Riley 1992 | Well-trained runners (18 M) | Dose: 3 g of coffee (150-200 mg of caffeine) Timing: 60 min pre-event | 1,500 m race on treadmill | Yes | Mean 1,500 time improved by ~4.2 s ($p < .05$) with caffeine compared with placebo. |
| Wiles et al. 1992 | Well-trained runners (10 M) | Dose: 3 g of coffee (150-200 mg of caffeine) Timing: 60 min pre-event | 1,500 m race: 1.1 km at constant speed + 1 min self-selected final burst | Yes | Caffeine increased speed during 1 min final burst by ~0.6 km/hr, equivalent to 10 m ($p < .05$). |
| CROSS-COUNTRY SKIING | | | | | |
| Stadheim et al. 2013 | Highly trained cross-country skiers (10 M) | Dose: 6 mg/kg Timing: 75 min pre-event | 8 km double poling ergometer time trial | Yes | Caffeine ingestion improved performance by 4% with a reduction in times to complete the 8 km TT from 34:26±1:25 to 33:01±1:24 min (p= 0.003). Novelty of study was focus on performance in which speed is generated by small muscle mass of arms. |
| ROWING | | | | | |
| Carr, Gore, and Dawson 2011 | Well-trained rowers (8 M) | Dose: 6 mg/kg Timing: 60 min pre-event Note: Study also involved arms with bicarbonate and caffeine + bicarbonate. | 2,000 m ergometer row | Yes | Caffeine enhanced ergometer mean power by ~2%: 354 ± 67 W vs. 346 ± 61 W with placebo. However, bicarbonate reduced performance by a similar amount due to gastrointestinal effects. |
| Skinner et al. 2010 | Competitive rowers (10 M) | Dose: 2, 4, or 6 mg/kg Timing: 60 min pre-event | 2,000 m ergometer row | No | Wide variability in plasma caffeine and performance response among individuals. |

*(continued)*

**Table 5.3** *(continued)*

| Study | Subjects[a] | Caffeine intake | Measurement of sports performance | Was it enhanced? | Technical comments |
|---|---|---|---|---|---|
| | | | ROWING *(continued)* | | |
| Bruce et al. 2000 | Well-trained rowers (8 M) | Dose: 6 mg/kg or 9 mg/kg Timing: 60 min pre-event | 2,000 m ergometer row | Yes for both doses | Compared with placebo, caffeine trial was faster by 1.3% for 6 mg/kg dose and 1% for 9 mg/kg dose ($p < .05$). Some participants had urinary caffeine concentrations above 12 µg/ml with the higher caffeine dose. |
| Anderson et al. 2000 | Well-trained rowers (8 F) | Dose: 6 mg/kg or 9 mg/kg Timing: 60 min pre-event | 2,000 m ergometer row | Yes for both doses | Compared with placebo, caffeine trial was faster by 0.7% and 1.3% for 6 mg/kg and 9 mg/kg doses, respectively ($p < .05$). Performance improvement was achieved primarily by enhancing the first 500 m of rowing. |
| | | | SWIMMING | | |
| Burke et al. (submitted for publication) | Elite and highly trained swimmers (7M, 8F) | Dose: 2 mg/kg Timing: 60 min pre-event | 100 m race (best stroke) | No, but RPE were lower | No difference in reaction time, 50 m split, or 100 m race time between trials; however, RPE was lower in the caffeine trial ($p = .01$). Self-reports found that caffeine typically increased the time taken to fall asleep after the trial and reduced the quality of sleep. |
| Vandenbogaerde and Hopkins 2010 | 9 competitive swimmers (6M, 3F) | Doses: varying up to 5 mg/kg Timing: 75 min pre-event Note: Study design involved mixed modeling of 2-8 training TTs and 2-7 race swims with various interventions of caffeine, placebo, and time of day. Swimmers performed their main events, which differed in stroke and distance. | 100-400 m TT or race according to individuals' main event of stroke and distance | Yes | 100 mg caffeine enhanced performance in 1 min training and competition TTs by 1.3% (large effect; 90% CI = 0.3%-2.8% and 0.1%-2.6%, respectively). Each additional 100 mg caffeine reduced the benefit slightly by 0.1% (unclear; 90% CI = 0.5%-0.3%). The effect of a doubling of TT time on the effect of caffeine was 0.3% (unclear; 90% CI = 1.5%-0.9%). The placebo effect was a slight improvement of 0.2% (unclear; 90% CI = 1.0%-1.4%). Caffeine also had small effects in increasing focus, decreasing length of sleep, and increasing time to fall to sleep. |
| Pruscino et al. 2008 | Elite swimmers (6 M) | Dose: 6.2 mg/kg Timing: 45 min before race 1 Note: Study also involved arms with bicarbonate and caffeine + bicarbonate. | 2 × 200 m freestyle races separated by 30 min | Race 1: Perhaps Race 2: No, perhaps even slower | Compared with placebo trial, caffeine improved performance by 1% in first swim (2:02.42 ± 3.17 vs. 2:03.77 ± 3.21 m:s for caffeine vs. placebo) but caused a trend to greater drop-off in second swim (1.2% ± 0.7% vs. 0.4% ± 0.7% slower). Bicarbonate appeared to counteract this drop-off. Small sample size makes interpretation difficult. |
| MacIntosh and Wright 1995 | Well-trained swimmers (7M, 4F) | Dose: 6 mg/kg Timing: 60 min prerace | 1,500 m freestyle race | Yes | 23 s improvement in swimming time with caffeine ($p < .05$). |

| Study | Subjects[a] | Caffeine intake | Measurement of sports performance | Was it enhanced? | Technical comments |
|---|---|---|---|---|---|
| Collomp et al. 1992 | Well-trained swimmers (3M, 4F) | Dose: 250 mg (~4 mg/kg) Timing: 60 min before race 1 | 2 × 100 m swimming races separated by 20 min | Yes | Caffeine increased swimming velocity in both races ($p < .01$) and prevented the decrease in velocity otherwise seen in the second swim with the placebo treatment. |
| CYCLING | | | | | |
| Astorino et al. 2012b | Endurance-trained cyclists, triathletes, runners (9 M, F) | Dose: 5 mg/kg Timing: 60 min pre-event 2 caffeine trials plus 1 placebo trial | 10 km TT | Yes | Caffeine enhanced performance by 1.6% (trial 1 = 16.98 ± 0.96 min) and 1.9% (trial 2 = 16.92 ± 0.97 min) compared with placebo trial (17.25 ± 0.96 min), $p < .05$. Individual differences in responses to caffeine were demonstrated, with 2 of the 9 subjects showing a consistent failure to improve performance. |
| Jenkins et al. 2008 | Trained cyclists (13 M) | Dose • 1 mg/kg • 2 mg/kg • 3 mg/kg Timing: 60 min pre-event | 15 min cycling at 60% $\dot{V}O_2$max + 15 min TT | No for 1 mg/kg Yes for 2 mg/kg Yes for 3 mg/kg | Work done during the 15 min TT was increased by 4% (1.0%-6.8%) with 2 mg/kg dose and 3% (−0.4%-6.8%) with 3 mg/kg dose. Performance improvement varied in magnitude among individuals. |
| TRACK CYCLING | | | | | |
| Kilding, Overton, and Gleave 2012 | Well-trained cyclists (10 M) | Dose: 3 mg/kg Timing: 60 min pre-event Note: Study also involved arms with bicarbonate and caffeine + bicarbonate. | 3 km TT | Yes | Caffeine increased power output by 2.4% and reduced TT time by 0.9% (both deemed to be of practical importance and statistical significance). A similar improvement was achieved with bicarbonate supplementation in a separate trial, but the combination of the two supplements did not further enhance the performance benefits over each supplement used separately. |
| Paton, Lowe, and Irvine 2010 | Competitive cyclists (9 M) | Dose: 240 mg Timing: During break between blocks 2 and 3 Caffeine provided as caffeinated gum with rapid absorption. | 4 blocks of repeated sprints Each block: 5 × 30 s | Yes | Caffeine attenuated fatigue in the second sets of sprints. Mean power in the second 10 sprints was reduced by 5.8% in placebo trial but only 0.4% in caffeine trial. Results suggest caffeine would provide a worthwhile performance enhancement for repeated sprints during a road race, criterium, or mass-start track race. |
| Wiles, Coleman, Tegerdine, and Swaine 2006 | Trained cyclists (8M) | Dose: 5 mg/kg Timing: 75 min pre-event | 1 km cycling TT | Yes | Caffeine race was faster by 2.4 s or 3.1% (95% CI = 0.7%-5.6%) ($p < .05$), which also achieved practical significance in real-life kilo track cycling event. |

[a]Unless otherwise stated, all studies used a crossover design in which subjects acted as their own controls, undertaking both the caffeine and placebo trial; TT = time trial. M = males, F = females. RPE = ratings of perceived effort

**Table 5.4** Does Caffeine Enhance the Performance of Stop-and-Go Sports?

| Study | Subjects[a] | Caffeine intake | Measurement of sports performance | Was it enhanced? | Technical comments |
|---|---|---|---|---|---|
| TEAM SPORTS | | | | | |
| Tucker et al. 2013 | Provincial-level basketball players (5 M) | Dose: 3 mg/kg Timing: 60 min pre-event | Incremental treadmill test to exhaustion + 10 vertical rebound jumps | No | No change in aerobic capacity or reactive strength index (height jumped/hang time) with caffeine intake. |
| Bassini et al. 2013 | Professional soccer players (19 M) Study was undertaken with a parallel group design in which subjects were divided into two groups | Dose: 3 mg/kg Timing: 60 min pre-event On the basis of their plasma caffeine response to caffeine ingestion, the caffeine group was further divided into high responders and low responders | 90 min variable distance run + YoYo Intermittent Recovery Test level 2 *Carbohydrate consumed during exercise protocol* | No | Caffeine supplementation did not significantly affect the performance of the YoYo test (No caffeine = 12.3 ± 0.3 km·h, 1449 ± 378 m; Low responder caffeine = 12.2 ± 0.5 km·h, 1540 ± 630 m; High responder caffeine = 12.3 ± 0.5 km·h, 1367 ± 330 m). |
| Del Coso et al. 2013 | National level Rugby 7 players (16 F) | Dose: 3 mg/kg Timing: 60 min pre-event Caffeine provided as energy drink with placebo as decaffeinated energy drink | Field study<br>• 15-s maximal jump<br>• 6 × 30 m sprint test,<br>• 3 x rugby sevens games against another national team (GPS monitoring) | Yes<br><br>No<br><br>Yes | Testing prior to games showed that the energy drink increased muscle power output during the jump series (23.5 ± 10.1 vs. 25.6 ± 11.8 kW, $p = .05$) but did not affect maximal running speed during the repeated sprint test (25.0 ± 1.5 vs. 25.0 ± 1.7 km/h). Individual running pace and instantaneous speed during the games were assessed using global positioning satellite (GPS) devices and showed an increase in running pace during the games (87.5 ± 8.3 vs. 95.4 ± 12.7 m/min, $p < .05$) and pace at sprint velocity (4.6 ± 3.3 vs. 6.1 ± 3.4 m/min, $p < .05$). The ingestion of the energy drink resulted in a higher post-competition urine caffeine concentration than the placebo (3.3 ± 0.7 vs. 0.2 ± 0.1 µg/mL; $p < .05$). |

| Study | Subjects[a] | Caffeine intake | Measurement of sports performance | Was it enhanced? | Technical comments |
|---|---|---|---|---|---|
| Astorino et al. 2012c | Collegiate soccer players (15 F) | Dose: 1.3 mg/kg Timing: 60 min pre-event Caffeine provided as energy drink | | No | Mean sprint time was similar ($p > .05$) between Red Bull (11.31±0.61 s) and placebo (11.35±0.61 s). HR and RPE increased ($p < .05$) during the bouts, but there was no effect ($p > .05$) of Red Bull on either variable versus placebo. |
| Duncan, Taylor, and Lyons 2012 | National-level hockey players (13 M) | Dose: 5 mg/kg Timing: 60 min pre-event 3 trials: 1 × rested and 2 × fatigued (following 1 min of repeated squat thrusts) with either placebo or caffeine treatment | Hockey slalom sprint dribble test (30 m dribble around cones) Chapman stick-handling test (measuring ball control) *Protocol too brief to require intake during exercise* | Yes Yes | Fatigue treatment reduced sprint dribble test time and ball-handling scores, but these effects were partially rescued by caffeine treatment. Caffeine reduced RPE and increased readiness to invest physical and mental effort in fatigue trials. |
| Spradley et al. 2012 | Recreationally active subjects (12 M) | Dose: 300 mg caffeine Timing: 20 min pre-event Caffeine provided as preworkout supplement containing branched-chain amino acids (BCAAs), beta-alanine, and citrulline malate. | 2 h protocol involving repetition of tests of • reaction and agility • critical velocity • repeated leg press (75% 1RM) *Water consumed during exercise protocol* | Yes No Yes | Caffeine trial associated with an improvement in muscular endurance and reaction/agility tests via a reduction in fatigue seen throughout the protocol. No change in critical velocity outcomes. |
| Gwacham and Wagner 2012 | Division 1 American football players (20 M) | Dose: 120 mg (~1.2 mg/kg) in energy drink Timing: 35 min before warm-up (i.e., 60 min before performance test) Caffeine consumed as low-calorie energy drink that also contained 200 mg taurine and other ingredients. | RAST (Running-based Anaerobic Sprint Test) involving 6 × 35 m sprints with 10 s recovery *Protocol too brief to require intake during exercise* | No | Sprint times became progressively slower over the test, regardless of caffeine supplementation. Though there was no overall effect of caffeine across the whole group of players, the researchers suggested a relationship between the effect of caffeine supplementation and habitual caffeine use, with the players who usually consumed the least amount of caffeine showing a better average sprint time in the caffeine trial. However, they acknowledge their method of ascertaining usual caffeine intake may not be reliable. |

*(continued)*

**Table 5.4** *(continued)*

| Study | Subjects[a] | Caffeine intake | Measurement of sports performance | Was it enhanced? | Technical comments |
|---|---|---|---|---|---|
| **TEAM SPORTS** *(continued)* | | | | | |
| Del Coso, Muñoz-Fernández, et al. 2012a | Semipro-fessional soccer players (19 M) | Dose: 3 mg/kg<br>Timing: 60 min pre-event<br>Caffeine consumed as low-calorie energy drink that also contained 200 mg taurine and other ingredients. | Field study<br>15 s maximal height jump +<br>7 × 30 s repeated sprint test (30 s recovery) +<br>2 × 40 min game with 15 min halftime break<br><br>*Information on intake during game not provided* | Yes<br><br>Yes<br><br><br>Yes | GPS coverage of games showed that the caffeinated drink was associated with a longer distance covered in the match (7782 ± 878 vs. 7352 ± 881, $p < .05$, effect size = 0.48), with greater amounts covered at medium-intensity, high-intensity, and sprinting paces and less covered by walking. The number of sprints was also greater (30 ± 10 vs. 24 ± 8, $p < .05$, ES = 0.75). Pregame tests showed greater average jump height (35.8 ± 5.5 cm vs. 34.7 ± 4.7, $p < .05$, ES = 0.23) and power generated during the jump test with the caffeine trial. Similarly, greater mean peak running speed was achieved during the repeated sprint test with the caffeine trial (26.3 ± 1.8 vs. 25.6 ± 2.1 km/h, $p < .05$, ES = 0.33). 17 of 19 players were considered to be responders to caffeine, showing a performance improvement with at least 2 of the 3 tests; 2 players were deemed to be non-responders. |
| Duvnjak-Zaknich, Dawson, Wallman, and Henry 2011 | Moderately trained team players (10 M) | Dose: 6 mg/kg<br>Timing: 60 min pregame | 80 min (4 × 20 min) simulated team sport running test (9,360 m) with agility tests pregame, at the end of each quarter<br>• Total time<br>• Reactive agility time<br>• Decision time<br>• Movement time<br>• Decision-making accuracy<br><br>*Water consumed during exercise protocol* | <br><br><br><br><br><br>Yes<br>Yes<br><br>Yes<br>Yes<br>Perhaps | Compared with placebo trial, results for caffeine trial were consistently faster for total time (2.3%), reactive agility time (3.9%), movement time (2.7%), and decision time (9.3%) ($p < .05$). These faster times were supported by qualitative analyses of "likely" to "almost certain benefit" and moderate to large effect sizes at various testing times for total time, reactive agility time, and movement time. Effect of caffeine on decision time at different testing times was less clear. Improved decision-making accuracy (3.8%) after caffeine inges-tion was supported by a likely benefit (quarter 1) and large effect sizes (quarters 1 and 4). |

| Study | Subjects[a] | Caffeine intake | Measurement of sports performance | Was it enhanced? | Technical comments |
|---|---|---|---|---|---|
| Roberts et al. 2010 | University-level rugby union forwards (8 M) | Dose: 4 mg/kg Timing: 60 min pregame 3 trials: caffeine + carbohydrate, carbohydrate, placebo | Bath University Rugby Shuttle Test (BURST): $4 \times 21$ min blocks, with each block involving 5 cycles of intermittent movement and rugby tasks with performance test and 15 m at the end of each cycle and motor skills at the end of each block<br>• Performance test<br>• 15 m sprint<br>• Motor skills<br><br>*Carbohydrate consumed during some exercise protocols* | Perhaps<br>Yes<br>Yes | Performance measures declined across the trial with placebo treatment. Carbohydrate alone did not reduce this decline. However, analysis using practical significance curves showed that the caffeine and carbohydrate trial resulted in a likely improvement for maximal intensity performance test: There was a 98% chance of a 2% improvement. The 15 m sprint test and motor skills test were faster with caffeine and carbohydrate than placebo trial ($p < .05$). RPE was lower in caffeine plus carbohydrate. |
| Gant, Ali, and Foskett 2010 | Premier-grade soccer players (15 M) | Dose: 3.7 mg/kg Timing: 60 min pregame + 15 min intervals during the event | 90 min ($6 \times 15$ min) simulated soccer running test (LIST) with skills test (LPST) measured pretrial and during the 6 breaks<br>• Sprint time<br>• Countermovement jump (CMJ)<br>• LPST = movement time + penalty time<br><br>*Carbohydrate consumed before and during exercise protocol* | Yes<br>Yes<br>No | 15 m sprint performance deteriorated over time in both trials but was attenuated by caffeine supplementation such that sprints were faster over the last 3 blocks of sprints. Decrease in performance of CMJ over time was prevented with caffeine. There was no difference in LPST outcomes between trials. There also was no difference in RPE between trials, meaning that players produced more work for the same perceived effort with caffeine intake. Caffeine also increased subjects' rating of pleasure. |
| Foskett et al. 2009 | Soccer players (12 M) | Dose: 6 mg/kg Timing: 60 min pregame | 90 min ($6 \times 15$ min) simulated soccer running test (LIST test) with skills test (LPST) measured pretrial and during the 6 breaks<br>• Sprint time<br>• Countermovement jump (CMJ)<br>• LPST = movement time + penalty time<br><br>*Water consumed during exercise protocol* | No<br>Yes<br>Yes | 15 m sprint performance deteriorated over time but was not changed by caffeine supplementation. LSPT test involves combination of passing accuracy, dribbling ability, recognition, and response to visual and audible stimuli, with score being summed from movement time less penalty time (for errors). LSPT was enhanced in caffeine trial by 4% ($p < .05$), with improvement solely due to 20% reduction in penalties (errors). Urinary caffeine concentrations remained below 12 µg/ml in all subjects. |

*(continued)*

**Table 5.4** *(continued)*

| Study | Subjects[a] | Caffeine intake | Measurement of sports performance | Was it enhanced? | Technical comments |
|---|---|---|---|---|---|
| | | | **TEAM SPORTS** *(continued)* | | |
| Carr et al. 2008 | Team athletes (10 M) | Dose: 6 mg/kg Timing: 60 min pre-event | • 5 sets of 6 × 20 m sprints with 180% turn at 10 m <br>  • Sets 1, 3, 5 on 25 s repeats <br>  • Sets 2, 4 on 60 s repeat <br>• 3 × reaction tests before and after sprints <br><br>*Protocol too brief for intake during exercise* | Yes <br><br><br><br><br><br>Perhaps | Caffeine enhanced sprint time overall compared with placebo, with effects seen particularly in sets 2 and 3; total time for sets 1, 3, 5 with short recovery was improved by 1.5 s ($p < .05$), while total time for sets 2 and 4 improved 0.8 sec ($p < .05$). Reaction times were faster in postsprint tests; there was a trend (moderate effect size) to better reaction time on caffeine trial. |
| Glaister et al. 2008 | College students involved in team sports (21 M) | Dose: 5 mg/kg Timing: 60 min pre-event | 12 × 30 m running sprints repeated at 35 s interval <br><br>*Protocol too brief to require intake during exercise* | Yes | Caffeine resulted in a 0.06 ± 0.05 s reduction in fastest 30 m sprint time (95% likely range = 0.04-0.09 s) over first three sprints, but this was offset by a 1.2 ± 1.7% increase (5.9 ± 2.9% vs. 4.6 ± 1.8%) in fatigue (95% likely range = 0.3%-2.2%) over the sprint series. |
| Stuart, Hopkins, Cook, and Cairns 2006 | Rugby union players (9 M) | Dose: 6 mg/kg Timing: 70 min pregame | Simulated rugby union protocol: 2 × 40 min circuits involving repetitions of the following: <br>• 20 m sprint speed <br>• 30 m sprint speed <br>• Offensive sprint <br>• Defensive sprint <br>• Drive 1 power <br>• Drive 2 power <br><br>• Tackle speed <br>• Passing ability <br><br>*Water consumed during exercise protocol* | <br><br><br><br><br>Possible <br>Very likely <br>Likely <br>Likely <br>Likely <br>No; possible harm <br>Likely <br>Likely | Study involved magnitude-based inferences rather than traditional statistics to examine the results. Compared with a placebo trial, caffeine caused improvements of 0.5%-3% in performance of sprint tasks, with a greater improvement in second half, presumably due to a reduction in fatigue. There was also a 10% improvement in ability to pass the ball accurately because of enhancement of arousal or attention. One test (second power drive) showed a possible impairment of performance. |
| Schneiker, Bishop, Dawson, and Hackett 2006 | Team athletes (10 M) | Dose: 6 mg/kg Timing: 60 min pregame | 2 × 36 min cycle protocol, each involving 18 × 4 s sprint with 2 min recovery | Yes | Total work during sprints in first half was 8.5% greater in caffeine trial than placebo, and work in second half was 7.6% greater in caffeine trial (both $p < .05$). Mean peak power scores achieved during sprints in first and second halves were 7% and 6.6% greater in caffeine trial than placebo (both $p < .05$). |

| Study | Subjects[a] | Caffeine intake | Measurement of sports performance | Was it enhanced? | Technical comments |
|---|---|---|---|---|---|
| Paton, Hopkins, and Volle-bregt 2001 | Team athletes (16 M) | Dose: 6 mg/kg<br>Timing: 60 min pregame | $10 \times 20$ m running sprints on interval of 10 s<br><br>*Protocol too brief to require intake during exercise* | No | Negligible difference between caffeine and placebo trials for time to complete 10 sprints and decay in performance over 10 sprints. |
| | | | RACKET SPORTS | | |
| Klein et al. 2012 | US college tennis players (8 F, 8 M) | Dose: 6 mg/kg<br>Timing: 60 min pregame | 45 min intermittent treadmill run to mimic intensities of game play +<br>Tennis skill test (stroke accuracy) | Test | Caffeine improved the number of successful shots during the Tennis Skill Test (2.1%; caffeine=295±11 shots; placebo=289±10 shots, $p < .05$), but performance was not influenced by the genotype. Subjects were divided into groups based on differences in their expression of the *CYP1A2* gene (involved in caffeine metabolism). There was a strong trend for individuals with an AA expression of this gene (n = 7) to increase heart rate after caffeine intake but not the individuals with C alleles (n = 9). Nevertheless, both groups improved tennis performance. This provides preliminary support for a greater physiological effect of caffeine in people with a certain genetic makeup, though this had no apparent influence on tennis performance. |
| Hornery et al. 2007 | Highly trained tennis players (12 M) | Dose: 3 mg/kg<br>Timing: 60 min pregame | Simulated tennis match (2 h 40 min) against a ball machine<br>• Stroke velocity<br>• Stroke accuracy<br>• Serve kinematics<br>• Tennis-specific perceptual skill | <br><br><br>No<br>No<br>Yes<br>No | Tennis skills declined over time. Caffeine reduced the loss of serving velocity in the last set ($p < .05$). Other strategies also tested in other trials in this study (precooling and carbohydrate intake) reduced physiological stress but did not reduce the decay in performance over time. |

*(continued)*

**Table 5.4** *(continued)*

| Study | Subjects[a] | Caffeine intake | Measurement of sports performance | Was it enhanced? | Technical comments |
|---|---|---|---|---|---|
| RACKET SPORTS *(continued)* | | | | | |
| Strecker et al. 2007 | Collegiate tennis players (10 M) | Dose: 3 mg/kg Timing: 90 min pregame | Skill test performed before, 30 min later, 60 min later, and after 90 min of simulated tennis play against a ball machine—15 ground strokes in all 4 directions (60 shots total)<br>• Forehand cross-court<br>• Forehand up the line<br>• Backhand cross-court<br>• Backhand up the line | <br><br><br><br><br><br><br><br><br>Yes<br><br>Yes<br><br>No<br><br>No | Caffeine trial showed better performance of both forehand shots across the 90 min of simulated tennis play. There was no difference in skill in backhand shots between trials. |
| Vergauwen, Brouns, and Hespel 1998 | Well-trained tennis players (13 M) | Dose and timing: 5 mg/kg 1 h pregame + 0.75 mg/kg per hour over 2 h Separate trials for caffeine + carbohydrate, carbohydrate only, and placebo | Tests undertaken before and after 2 h match play<br>• Skill test (Leuven Tennis Performance Test) measuring stroke quality<br>• 70 m shuttle run<br><br>*Carbohydrate or water consumed according to trial* | <br><br>No<br><br><br><br>No | Carbohydrate trial resulted in maintenance of stroke quality and shuttle run speed, whereas placebo trial resulted in deterioration of these aspects of performance. Caffeine added to carbohydrate did not further enhance posttrial performance. The researchers suggest that the caffeine dose was too high. However, it is also possible that the effect could only be expected if the protocol had caused fatigue, which did not occur because of carbohydrate intake. |
| Ferrauti, Weber, and Struder 1997 | Competitive tennis players (8 M, 8 F) | 364 mg for males 260 mg for females (~4-4.5 mg/kg) | 4 h tennis singles play (with 30 min break after 150 min) Tests of skill and speed undertaken at end of 4 h:<br>• 6 × 15 min sprint with 30 min rest<br>• Hitting accuracy and success during games | <br><br><br><br><br>No<br><br>Yes for females; no for males | No effect of caffeine supplementation on tennis-specific running speed, hitting accuracy, or success of games played during 4 h with male participants. However, female players had greater success during tennis play in caffeine trial than placebo. |
| COMBAT SPORTS | | | | | |
| Souissi et al. 2012 | Highly trained judoka (judoists) (12 M) | Dose: 5 mg/kg Timing: 60 min pre-event | Cycling: 30 s Wingate test Reaction time | Yes Yes | Caffeine increased vigor and anxiety in Profile of Mood States (POMS) test. Reaction time improved (reduced time to react to stimuli) with caffeine intake. Caffeine increased mean power and peak power in cycling test but did not change fatigue index. |

[a]Unless otherwise stated, all studies used a crossover design in which subjects acted as their own controls, undertaking both the caffeine and placebo trial; TT = time trial. M = males, F = females

**Table 5.5** Does Caffeine Enhance Performance of Strength and Power Events (Throws, Lifts, and Sprints)?

| Study | Subjects[a] | Caffeine intake | Measurement of sports performance | Was it enhanced? | Technical comments |
|---|---|---|---|---|---|
| Glaister et al. 2012 | Resistance-trained subjects (17 M) | Dose: 2, 4, 6, 8 and 10 mg/kg Timing: 6 min pre-event | 10 s cycling sprint | No | Caffeine had no effect at any dose on peak power, mean power, or time to reach peak power. |
| Del Coso, Salinero, et al. 2012 | Active subjects (9 M, 3 F) | Dose: 1 and 3 mg/kg Timing: 60 min pre-event Caffeine provided as energy drink with taurine and L-carnitine. | Half squat Bench press | Yes for 3 mg/kg No for 1 mg/kg | Maximal power output increased by ~7% in both half squat and bench press with higher caffeine dose but no low dose. High dose also caused increase in caffeine side effects (i.e., increase in heart rate and blood pressure, gut upset). |
| Eckerson et al. 2012 | Resistance-trained subjects (17 M) | Dose: 160 mg Timing: 60 min pre-event Caffeine provided as low-calorie energy drink with 2,000 mg taurine or as same energy drink without taurine. Delete whole remnant | 1RM bench press | No | Neither the energy drink nor the caffeine-only version had any effect on 1RM for bench press compared with placebo (115.13 ± 16.19 kg, 114.87 ± 16.16 kg, and 114.07 ± 16.09 kg, respectively). There was also no effect on muscular endurance (repetitions to failure) at 70% 1RM. |
| Bellar et al. 2012 | Well-trained throwers (shot put) (4M, 5F) | Dose: 100 mg Timing: 5 min pre-event Caffeine provided as caffeinated chewing gum, allowing rapid mouth absorption of caffeine. | 6 × shot-put throws separated by 1 min | Yes for first throw and trend to overall | Caffeine was associated with higher scores on a reaction time test both at the beginning and the end of the session. Caffeine also achieved rapider and greater consistency with throw distance compared with placebo trial. |
| Goldstein, Jacobs, et al. 2010 | Resistance trained (15 F) | Dose: 6 mg/kg Timing: 60 min pre-event | 1RM bench press | Yes | Caffeine enhanced strength for 1RM for bench press. |
| Williams et al. 2008 | Resistance trained (9 M) | Dose: 300 mg (~3.6. mg/kg) Timing: 45 min pre-event | 1RM bench press 1RM lat pull-down | No No | Athletes reported higher mood and alertness with caffeine, but this did not translate into enhanced strength. |
| Astorino, Rohmann, and Firth 2008 | Resistance trained (22 M) | Dose: 6 mg/kg Timing: 60 min pre-event | 1RM bench press 1RM leg press | No No | No changes in strength of lower or upper body with caffeine. |
| Beck et al. 2006 | Resistance trained (37 M) Parallel group design— trials 48 h apart | Dose: 6 mg/kg Timing: 60 min pre-event | 1RM bench press 1RM leg extension | Yes No | Caffeine-supplement group showed a 2% (2 kg) increase in upper-body strength (bench press 1RM max) following treatment, but no change in placebo group. There were no differences in lower-body strength in either group. |

[a] Unless otherwise stated, all studies used a crossover design in which subjects acted as their own controls, undertaking both the caffeine and placebo trial; RM = Repetition maximum (the highest load that can be lifted once). M = males, F = females

**Table 5.6.** Does Caffeine Enhance Performance of Skill Sports (Golf, Archery, Shooting)?

| Study | Subjects[a] | Caffeine intake | Measurement of sports performance | Was it enhanced? | Technical comments |
|---|---|---|---|---|---|
| Cunningham (unpublished data cited in Share et al. 2009) | Elite archers | Dose:<br>• 2 mg/kg<br>• 6 mg/kg<br>Timing: 60 min pre-event | 72 arrow round competition | Perhaps for 2mg/kg<br>No for 6 mg/kg | Score improved by 5.7 points (meaningful but not statistically significant) for the lower caffeine dose but decreased by 7.7 points with the higher dose. |
| Share et al. 2009 | Elite double-trap shooters (7 M) | Dose:<br>• 2 mg/kg<br>• 4 mg/kg<br>Timing: 60 min pre-event | Shooting: 4 rounds × 50 shots<br>• Shooting accuracy<br>• Reaction time<br>• Target tracking times | No<br><br>No<br>No | There were no differences over time with shooting parameters and no differences between caffeine trials and placebo. |
| Stevenson et al. 2009 | Experienced golfers—handicap ~15 (20 M) | Dose: 1.6 mg/kg (in sport drink)<br>Timing: immediately pregame and at holes 6 and 12 of simulated 18-hole golf game | Simulated golf game—18 holes with testing at each hole<br>• 5 m putt<br>• 2 m putt<br>• Mood (every 3 holes) | Yes<br>Yes<br>Yes | Putting ability and alertness were improved by caffeine, while the increased perceptions of fatigue that occurred over time were reduced. Note: Caffeine was consumed in combination with carbohydrate, so effects from each source can't be separated in present study design. |

[a] Unless otherwise stated, all studies used a crossover design in which subjects acted as their own controls, undertaking both the caffeine and placebo trial; M = males, F = females

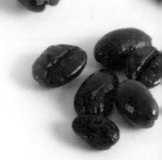

# Chapter
· · · · · · · · · · · · ·
# 6

# Known Side Effects, Health Risks, and Cautions

Caffeine use in all populations, including athletes, needs to be viewed against the backdrop of its effects on human health. It has been suggested that moderate daily caffeine intakes of up to 400 mg over the course of a day (6 mg/kg) are not associated with adverse effects in healthy populations. Indeed, it could be argued that the world has become a giant test tube, with the sheer popularity of caffeine-containing beverages turning us all into subjects in an uncontrolled caffeine study. The results of this impromptu and changing experiment generally speak to the lack of serious health issues associated with typical caffeine intake patterns. Having said this, most countries have food and drug regulatory bodies that limit the number of foods and drinks that caffeine can be added to and the maximum amounts of caffeine that can be added. Some countries have also commissioned working groups to assess the safety aspects of dietary caffeine. In this chapter, we discuss possible concerns about caffeine use, especially in certain populations.

## Caffeine Can Be Lethal

We'll start with the worst-case scenario. People can—and have—died from caffeine overdoses, although these incidences are rare. A search of the literature indicates that deaths from caffeine intoxication or overdoses have appeared consistently for at least the last 30 years. One publication from 1980 reported that there had been seven previously documented cases. Many of these fatalities appeared to have occurred accidently when people consumed over-the-counter or nonprescription diet concoctions designed to suppress appetite where the main active ingredient was caffeine or in some cases a caffeine–ephedrine combination.

These caffeine-containing compounds are often called *look-alike drugs*, where people believe they are consuming diet-helper concoctions and are unaware of what is actually in the pills. In most cases they contain large amounts of caffeine.

It is important to understand just how much caffeine had to be taken by these people to lead to an overdose. We pointed out in chapter 2 that consuming 210, 420, and 630 mg of caffeine produced blood or plasma levels of 15 to 20 µM, 40 to 50 µM, and 60 to 75 µM (see figure 2.3). These amounts of caffeine amount to 3, 6, and 9 mg/kg for a 70 kg person, and it can be argued that 9 mg/kg is already a high dose. There are also a few experimental reports from some years ago where researchers gave 13 and 15 mg/kg, or about 910 to 1,050 mg of caffeine. With such high doses, blood caffeine could reach levels of 100 µM. It would be unlikely that an ethics research board would allow these levels of caffeine to be given to volunteers today.

How does this compare with blood caffeine levels reported in the case studies of caffeine overdose deaths? It is generally stated that blood levels greater than 500 µM are lethal, and in one report from 1985, documenting five cases of fatal caffeine overdoses, the blood levels ranged from 670 to 1,775 µM! In another case study of a death in 1989, the person's blood caffeine level was an astounding 8,000 µM, which is the by far the highest reported blood caffeine level ever. There is little direct information about just how much caffeine a person would have to take in order to reach these lethal levels, but it would have to be well over 5 g of caffeine. There are some cases of caffeine overdoses where the people have survived, including one case in which a 16-year-old male consumed 6 to 8 g of caffeine. His symptoms included extreme agitation, a high heart rate with many irregular beats, high levels of potassium and glucose in the blood, respiratory alkalosis from overbreathing, and chest pain. Other reported outcomes include vomiting, hallucinations, convulsions, and coma leading to death. The fact that a caffeine overdose normally causes vomiting is most likely a lifesaver because the excess caffeine is removed from the body and does not have a chance to enter the bloodstream.

I had an 80-kilogram swimmer at the Olympics take 600 mg of caffeine before a race—a double serving of a preworkout supplement. When I asked why and described the issues of overconsumption, the swimmer replied, "Yeah, but if you can control the buzz you will swim awesome." The swimmer subsequently swam well below the optimum, dying in the second half of the race because the athlete had gone out too hard. Obviously the swimmer wasn't able to control the buzz.

*Sports dietitian to elite athletes*

In recent years, there have continued to be case reports of caffeine fatalities, with one report in 2004 documenting four such cases and two more reported in a 2005 publication. In the latter study, blood samples revealed caffeine concentrations of 1,000 and 2,900 μM in the two individuals. Not surprisingly, there have been calls by the medical community to limit the sale of over-the-counter caffeine pills even though such products contain only 100 to 200 mg of caffeine and caffeine deaths are rare and are ruled as accidental.

Interestingly, an online resource has been developed to calculate excessive caffeine doses from drinks and foods. It allows a consumer to estimate the amounts of normal caffeine-containing products that are needed to reach the intakes considered lethal. Of course, this isn't a foolproof tool, and it shouldn't be used to encourage foolhardy intakes. However, it generally shows that it requires unlikely amounts of common products such as coffee or energy drinks to get into a toxic caffeine range. This resource is available at www.energyfiend.com.

## Energy Drinks: Why Do People Consume Them, and What Are the Side Effects?

To get a better feel for the background and outcomes of energy drinks, the emergency departments of two hospitals in San Diego surveyed 1,298 patients who came through their doors during 2009. The participants included Caucasians (48%), African Americans (17%), and Hispanics (18%), with ages ranging from 18 to 29 years (38%), 30 to 54 years (50%), and >55 years (12%). Reasons for consuming energy drinks included to increase energy (57%), to assist with the completion of work and study projects (10%), to help with prolonged stints of driving (2%), to enhance sports performance (2%), and to accompany alcohol intake (6%). A third of these patients reported adverse reactions or side effects from the energy drinks, including feeling shaky or jittery (22%) and suffering from insomnia (10%), heart palpitations (12%), gut upsets (6%), headaches (5%), chest pain (3%), and seizures (6 patients, representing less than .5%). Most of these issues were of mild to moderate concern, but some, such as the seizures, were serious. Equally concerning was the report that 6% of patients deliberately drank energy drinks while using illegal stimulants such as cocaine and methamphetamine. Although athletic use would appear to contribute only a minor part of the concern related to energy drinks, it is clear that other aspects of their use can be troubling in a small number of people.

## Side Effects and Risks

Normal amounts of caffeine-containing products, providing moderate to high caffeine doses (6-9 mg/kg or 420-630 mg), typically do not present any health risks. However, there are well-known side effects or adverse outcomes, including increased heart rate and sometimes small increases in blood pressure, anxiety, jitters, mental confusion, inability to focus, gastrointestinal unrest, insomnia, irritability, and what we call *blabbermouth syndrome*. It is common for a person to start talking, sometimes excessively, about 20 minutes after ingesting a large dose of caffeine. In one study in which subjects consumed caffeine doses of 9 and 13 mg/kg, the reported side effects were dizziness, headache, tremor, hunger sensations, insomnia, and diuresis (urine production).

Of course, caffeine-induced side effects vary considerably from person to person, as do the metabolic and performance effects. These side effects are not dangerous, but they can be disconcerting before training or competition. The side effects are much reduced at moderate doses of 4 to 5 mg/kg and most often not present at all at low doses of 3 mg/kg or less. Given the impressive development of recent evidence that athletic endurance and performance improve with low caffeine doses, it makes sense to recommend that they become the target for use in competitions after being experimented with in training.

Health concerns should also be considered for athletes who are habitual consumers of caffeine. Caffeine is a psychoactive substance, and if consumed daily, it can lead to a number of caffeine-use disorders, including caffeine intoxication, caffeine dependence and withdrawal syndrome, and caffeine-induced anxiety and sleep disorders. For example, people who consume moderate amounts of caffeine may experience withdrawal symptoms if they reduce their daily intake of caffeine. As discussed in chapter 9, the side effects of withdrawal include severe headaches, fatigue, lethargy, and flulike symptoms. These symptoms disappear rather quickly over time (2-4 days) and are rapidly reversed if caffeine is reintroduced. Of course, many caffeine consumers are so regular with their caffeine habits that they never experience withdrawal or reduced intakes. However, the lower the dose

I knew of a high-profile rugby player who played the worst game in his career when taking a high dose of caffeine (over 500 mg) for the first time, in the form of an over-the-counter tablet. The player reported hand tremors and feeling anxious and off his game. The most alarming negative effect was the heart palpitations, causing the player to fear he was having a heart attack. This influenced other players who then became reluctant to use caffeine in future matches.

*Sports dietitian to elite athletes*

of daily caffeine consumption and the lower the dose used before training and competition, the less likely it is that these symptoms will be present if caffeine is withdrawn.

## Mixing Caffeine With Other Stimulants

We know that caffeine is a mild CNS stimulant that can increase wakefulness, alertness, and vigilance. However, amphetamines and other stimulant drugs known as sympathomimetics are even more powerful stimulants and could produce dangerous effects when combined with caffeine. The most common mixture of caffeine with another stimulant has been the caffeine–ephedrine mix. Ephedrine is an amphetamine-like drug found in the herb ma huang, which was available as an over-the-counter product for many years. However, it is now banned from sales in most countries due to some well-documented overdoses and negative side effects. It is also a prohibited substance on the WADA banned list. However, there was a time when the caffeine–ephedrine mixture was commonly taken to suppress appetite and stimulate metabolism, promising increased fat use and weight loss among dieters and bodybuilders.

There was also much interest in this combination of stimulants in the military, where soldiers need to stay alert during missions and combat exercises. A series of studies from the Defence and Civil Institute of Environmental Medicine in Canada involving military recruits revealed that combinations of caffeine (5 mg/kg) and ephedrine (1 mg/kg) improved cycling endurance at ~85% $\dot{V}O_2$max and sprint cycling more than the individual ingredients alone did. However, about a quarter of the subjects experienced vomiting and nausea during high-intensity cycling. Reducing the caffeine dose to 4mg/kg and the ephedrine dose to 0.8 mg/kg preserved the performance benefits and reduced the side effects. Interestingly, when the exercise task was changed to a 10K run with backpack and helmet lasting about 45 minutes, the benefits of caffeine and ephedrine were not present.

However, the overriding point is that the caffeine–ephedrine combination often results in many side effects, including psychiatric and gastrointestinal symptoms, nausea, heart palpitations, and even death. Consequently, it is illegal in both the domestic and sporting worlds and should be avoided.

## Mixing Caffeine With Excessive Alcohol Use

Athletes normally are very disciplined people who carefully plan most aspects of what they do. But they also need downtime and like to party as much as (and sometimes more than) other people. The relationship between alcohol and caffeine used to be the search for a strong coffee brew as a pick-me-up after a late night of drinking or as an aid to sobering up. Now, however, it is common, especially among young people in party situations, to consume caffeine-containing products while they are consuming alcohol. In some countries, the combination of alcohol and caffeine exists in commercial products. However, the more typical scenario involves the self-mixing of energy drinks with alcoholic beverages such as spirits. The idea is that the uplifting and arousing effects of the energy drink counteract the depressant effects of alcohol, although in some cases people use the energy drinks to disguise the taste of the alcohol. Decreasing the subjective perceptions of being intoxicated may deliberately or inadvertently allow drinkers to increase their alcohol consumption.

The numerous constituents in energy drinks, such as taurine, ginseng, amino acids, inositol, ribose, and choline, have generally failed to show any active effects. This leaves the ingredients of interest in energy drinks as carbohydrate and caffeine. On the surface it may look as though an energy drink is optimal for energizing the muscles and the brain with its high carbohydrate content (9-15 g per 100 ml) and caffeine boost of 50 to 120 mg per serving. However, although the amount of caffeine added to many energy drinks is low to moderate and stated on the label, the total caffeine content of some drinks may not be specified due to the inclusion of other caffeine-containing compounds such as guarana, yerba maté, and kola nuts. The real concern comes when energy drinks are consumed in large volumes, which can easily happen if the athlete is determined to have a big session with alcohol and uses energy drinks as a mixer or chaser. There is already much concern regarding the dangers of excessive consumption of energy drinks due to their caffeine content, but the interaction with alcohol adds another dimension.

The literature is full of reports documenting the use of energy drinks along with alcohol. For example, studies from various countries have reported that 54% (United States), 25% to 40% (France), and 40% (Turkey) of college students consumed energy drinks with alcohol while partying, with many users reporting that they consumed at least three servings during the partying episodes (United States). The worry is that this type of behavior leads to a greater predisposition to alcohol dependence. However, a recent study from the Netherlands argues that a personality trait with higher levels of risk-taking behavior may be the primary reason for increased alcohol and drug abuse and that the co-consumption of energy drinks with alcohol is simply an expression of that type of lifestyle and personality. However, given the high prevalence of the co-consumption in young people, this explanation seems unlikely to account for the majority of people exhibiting this behavior.

# Caffeine, Coffee, Carbohydrate, and Type II Diabetes

When we eat carbohydrate-rich foods, they are absorbed into the blood as glucose, stimulating the pancreas gland to release insulin, which activates several tissues of the body (skeletal muscles, heart, adipose tissue) to take up the glucose and store it as glycogen or use it as fuel. There have been recent reports, however, demonstrating that when caffeine is consumed with a large amount of carbohydrate, it decreases the ability of the body to handle high blood glucose levels. This has been seen both in healthy men and in men who are obese or have type II diabetes. Because most of the glucose is normally taken up by the muscles (>75%), it appears that the caffeine is having a short-term antagonizing effect on the insulin-mediated glucose transport system in the muscles.

To confirm the suspicion of being diabetic or prediabetic, people take an oral glucose tolerance test (OGTT). This requires them to quickly drink a load of glucose (1 g/kg of their body mass) in a 250 ml drink, followed by the collection of blood samples every 15 to 20 min. This protocol is used to measure how quickly the glucose appears in the blood and, more importantly, how quickly it disappears into the tissues. Insulin, the hormone that helps the glucose transport process, is also measured to determine whether the person releases a normal amount of it. If the glucose is slow to be removed from the blood, then the person is prediabetic or diabetic. This is commonly seen in people who are physically inactive and obese.

Studies combining an OGTT with caffeine have been conducted with healthy, mildly active people who consumed a large dose of pure caffeine (~6 mg/kg, or ~420 mg for a 70 kg person) or caffeinated coffee. It is not clear whether the lower doses of caffeine, more typically consumed in a cup of coffee for instance, would have the same effect. It is also not known whether these effects would be present in an exercise-trained population or highly trained athletes.

> [Baseball player] Josh Hamilton returned to the Texas Rangers lineup on Monday night after an optometrist diagnosed the vision problem [ocular keratitis] that caused him to miss the past five games. . . . Doctors say high caffeine consumption can cause ocular keratitis. That might sound strange, but Hamilton wouldn't be the first baseball player to be told to cut back. Atlanta Braves catcher Brian McCann struggled with a mysterious and extended vision problem before decreasing his amount of caffeine consumption in 2010. Johnny Damon also cut caffeine while experiencing similar symptoms with the New York Yankees in 2009.
>
> *Kevin Kaduk (2012)*

Interestingly, and some would say paradoxically, the long-term consumption of coffee has been shown to be protective for type II diabetes—in other words, a lower risk of diabetes is found among people who are regular coffee consumers. This seems to be at odds with the acute effects of caffeine consumption on glucose disposal. However, the protective effects of coffee consumption are also seen in consumers of decaffeinated coffee, implying that the health effects of coffee must lie with other chemicals in it. Some possible explanations for the coffee-induced protection against diabetes include the effects of antioxidants present in coffee (especially the quinides). Coffee may also promote gut peptide hormones that are involved in satiety and the secretion of insulin and have prebiotic-like properties that favorably affect gut flora and digestion.

# General Health Issues and Epidemiology of Caffeine

There has been a longstanding concern that daily caffeine consumption may predispose people to an increased risk for a number of diseases. However, the overwhelming thread through all of the literature is that moderate caffeine consumption, defined as 400 mg/d or less, does not predispose people to increased disease risk. In fact, the studies that examine the relationship between caffeine consumption and all-cause mortality report either no relationship in men and women or report that caffeine was beneficial in reducing the risk of death, although this association is not strong in some studies. In one study that followed an elderly Finnish population for 14 years, the authors reported that the daily consumption of caffeine-containing coffee was inversely related with dying—good news!

# Caffeine and Heart Disease

Many studies and review articles have examined the effect of caffeine on cardiovascular health. The vast majority have concluded that the experimental findings do not support the hypothesis that caffeine or coffee consumption increases the risk of coronary heart disease, atherosclerosis, and stroke in healthy people or in people who already have type II diabetes or cardiovascular disease. Additional work suggests that the consumption of caffeinated coffee, decaffeinated coffee, or tea is not related to a greater incidence of rheumatoid arthritis, many forms of cancer, and liver disease. Two reports stated that coffee consumption may reduce liver cancer and chronic liver disease. So, the bottom line for those of us who consume moderate amounts of caffeine every day is that there is no concern for increased risk of the major diseases, and in some cases there appears to be a benefit.

Another line of concern involves the consumption of caffeine by people who already have forms of cardiac disease or are predisposed to heart arrhythmias. Caffeine has been publicized as a dangerous product for these people, and there is evidence from case reports that it may have a negative effect on existing problems of atrial fibrillation (the most common form of irregular heartbeat) in certain people. However, population-based studies do not support this as a widespread problem. There does not appear to be a link between a greater incidence of atrial fibrillation and caffeine consumption in healthy people, in people who have reported at least one episode of atrial fibrillation, or in people who have reported atrial fibrillation and have existing high blood pressure. In most cases, these studies reported that the daily caffeine consumption was moderate (<300-400 mg/kg). It does seem prudent, however, to recommend intakes below these moderate levels of caffeine for people with existing cardiovascular problems.

> The Cowboys don't prescribe or condone the use of No-Doz and Mason no longer uses it. However, six years ago he says No-Doz was all the rage at the Dogs. "I've been at clubs where they pump it into you," he says. "We won the comp [at Canterbury] on No-Doz. I think the whole NRL was taking them in 2004."
>
> *Rugby League player Willie Mason (Halloran, 2010)*

## Caffeine and Younger Athletes

Concerns over caffeine use by children target the immediate effects of caffeine on an immature body as well as the potential for long-term effects and habits. Little research has been done on the effects of caffeine in children—after all, it would be difficult to obtain ethical approval for many of these studies. Therefore, there is a lack of evidence related to caffeine and children, making it difficult to draw strong conclusions about the effects of caffeine on behavior, withdrawal symptoms, or long-term adverse health effects at various doses. However, there are earlier reports of increased anxiety in children at daily doses of 95 mg (~3 mg/kg) and reports suggesting adverse withdrawal effects associated with dietary caffeine in children. Typically, health authorities warn that children aged 12 or under should limit their daily caffeine intake to <2.5 mg/kg because of the increased risk of behavioral side effects.

As for the long-term implications, it is assumed that caffeine use in childhood lays the foundation for lifelong use, although this may not extend to caffeine abuse. There is some concern that many caffeinated products, such as energy drinks, are marketed directly to children and young adults. However, to date there are no data to conclude that caffeine consumption habits established early in life contribute to negative long-term health outcomes. There is also the worry that caffeine may become a gateway drug for young athletes, leading to the use of banned and more dangerous substances down the track. This has led to the argument that caffeine use should be discouraged in order to downplay the doping, win-at-all-costs mentality and set a proper example for young athletes. The Canadian Centre for Drug-Free Sport reported in 1993 that over 25% of youths aged 11 to 18 reported using caffeine in the previous year to help them do better in their athletic pursuits. This seems like a high number for young athletes but has been seen in other surveys as well.

We believe that it is inappropriate and unnecessary for children and young adults to consume caffeine as an ergogenic aid. Younger populations have the potential for greater performance enhancement through maturation and experience in their sport, along with adherence to proper training, nutrition, and recovery protocols. Until an athlete has matured and developed a sound foundation of good preparation habits, it is wasteful and inappropriate to look for shortcuts through ergogenic supplements.

## Caffeine and the Elderly

Studies of caffeine use by older people who are active have found evidence of many positive effects associated with staying active but also some negative outcomes. One large study examined a battery of performance and performance-related measures on 15 men and 15 women who were 70 years old or older. All the subjects in the study were healthy—the researchers rejected people who had various conditions or were taking medications that were deemed inappropriate or dangerous for participation in the study. The subjects abstained from caffeine for 48 hours and randomly received a caffeine dose equal to 6 mg/kg or a placebo. They repeated the study with the other treatment 1 week later. Caffeine increased plasma levels to ~55 μM, and it improved cycling endurance at 65% of maximal heart rate or ~55% of maximal oxygen uptake by 25% and isometric arm flexion endurance by 54%. The RPE—that is, the effort associated with the cycling—was reduced by 11%. However, caffeine had no effect on muscle strength, walking speed, and reaction and movement times. Finally, postural stability with eyes open was reduced by 25% with caffeine. Unfortunately, nearly half of the subjects picked the order of treatments, which may have affected their motivation in the tests. The authors also reported that 40% of the subjects did report some mild side effects of the caffeine, but nothing health related.

The bottom line is that if caffeine is taken around exercise, particularly when consumed at a lower dose and as part of normal dietary patterns, it helps to increase exercise tolerance and enjoyment. This might help some older people to stick with a good habit. There is also no reason to think that it wouldn't enhance performance in masters and veteran athletes, but event protocols should always be practiced.

## Caffeine and Pregnancy

Studies of a potential relationship between moderate caffeine consumption and reproductive health have failed to find consistent outcomes. Some studies have reported associations between caffeine intake and adverse reproductive outcomes such as premature births and babies with low birth weight, while others have not. The general consensus for all things related with pregnancy is to err on the side of caution, meaning that it is best not to consume moderate to large quantities of caffeine while pregnant.

## The Bottom Line

Various health agencies from countries around the world consider caffeine to be a generally safe compound, especially when daily consumption is low (80-250 mg or 1.1-3.5 mg/kg) or moderate (300-400 mg/d or 4-6 mg/kg). The use of caffeine by children carries greater risk, and children under the age of 12 are guided to limit daily caffeine intake to <2.5 mg/kg. Other special populations such as pregnant women and those with preexisting heart disease should also err with caution regarding their caffeine habits. Although extremely large doses of caffeine have been known to cause death, such events are rare. The most prevalent forms of unhealthy caffeine use appear to be chronically high intakes and mixing caffeine with other stimulants or excessive intakes of alcohol.

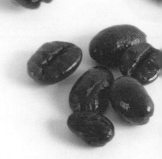

# Chapter

· · · · · · · · · · · · ·

# 7

# Permissibility of Caffeine Use in Sport

Exercise is an expression of physical activity, governed only by the limitations of the mind and the body. Sport, on the other hand, is highly governed by rules and regulations. Rules cover the duration, number of competitors, and playing space of an event; techniques and behavior on the field of play; codes of conduct for behavior away from the field of play; and the permissibility of ergogenic aids. Some rules are universal while others are specific to an event, a league, or an athlete or team. Antidoping rules apply to most sports or are at least monitored for the top group of competitors, with the most commonly applied antidoping code being the WADA code.

Other sporting organizations have official antidoping codes that are additional or parallel to the WADA code (e.g., the National Collegiate Athletic Association [NCAA] in the United States), and some club or sport governing bodies prepare codes of what is acceptable under their own auspices. For example, some sport clubs and institutes implement their own set of rules for what supplements are acceptable for players of certain ages or levels of sporting development. These rules are often set not only for the health and safety aspects but also to help younger athletes understand the priorities of getting the basics right. Caffeine often appears as one of the supplements deemed inappropriate for use by younger athletes or athletes who haven't reached a certain level of maturity in their sport.

Although in this chapter we deal with the position of caffeine in the official antidoping codes, we'll also see that the court of public opinion weighs in heavily on caffeine use. Caffeine has had a bumpy ride in its journey in the development of sport regulations, and even when the position on its use is clearly laid out, there is still confusion and debate.

# IOC Antidoping Programs (1968-2000)

The 1968 Winter Olympic Games in Grenoble saw the introduction of the first competition drug control program, organized under the jurisdiction of the IOC. This program involved the testing of a single urine sample collected after an event for the absence or presence of items described on a list of prohibited substances, as determined by the IOC Medical Commission. This list was developed with a focus on banning the use of stimulants and anabolic steroids. Caffeine was included on the list for the 1984 Los Angeles Summer Olympic Games, with the definition of a doping offense being urinary caffeine concentrations exceeding a cutoff of 15 µg/ml. In 1985, the threshold was reduced to 12 µg/ml.

The cutoff value was chosen to exclude normal or social coffee drinking and differentiate it from what was considered an unhealthy use of caffeine that was specifically consumed to enhance sports performance. A study by Belgian researchers, Drs Delbeke and Debackere, set out to establish what such excessive levels of caffeine would be. They examined urinary caffeine concentrations of 85 medium and strong coffee drinkers at random times of the day, then followed changes in urinary caffeine over 60 hours in a subgroup of these people. At the same time, they measured caffeine levels in urine samples provided by 775 cyclists at doping control during 1982.

Among the normal population, the researchers found mean values of urinary caffeine of 5.2 µg/ml, and they commented that normal levels were below 10 µg/ml while levels above 12.5 µg/ml were exceptional. Meanwhile, the doping-control study found ~650 cyclists who had detectable urinary caffeine levels, with a mean value of 3.4 µg/ml. From this, the researchers concluded that the caffeine levels in cyclists were lower than in the general population, although they noted that a subgroup of professional cyclists recorded a higher level of ~6 µg/ml. Nevertheless, only 1% of the samples were between 12.5 and 15 µg/ml and none was above 15 µg/ml. The final recommendations from the study were thus: "For all these reasons a urinary caffeine level above 10 µg/ml could be indicative of ingestion of caffeine with the intention of

The Broncos' victory was not without controversy. . . . Coaches from [other] teams noticed that some Boise State swimmers were drinking Red Bull energy drinks before their races. . . . [They] mounted a protest against Boise State because they thought the Broncos coaching staff and trainers were telling their athletes what to drink. "It's against NCAA rules for their trainers to administer that," Richmond said. "We protested that fact . . . but Boise State's coaches said they weren't the ones administering it. I just wanted to make sure the athletes were doing it on their own and it wasn't the coaches."

Juan López (2010)

improving physical performance. Nevertheless, we prefer to adopt a safety margin and propose a urinary caffeine limit of 15 μg/ml for sporting competitors" (Delbeke and Debackere, 1984, p. 182).

It is uncertain whether the IOC's 1984 decision on caffeine in sport was primarily related to safety concerns over very large doses of caffeine or the ethics of achieving performance advantages through caffeine use. In any case, over the next 15 years there were relatively few cases of positive doping outcomes for caffeine use among elite athletes. Some exceptions include high caffeine readings in race scenarios for former German world champion runner Inger Miller, South African Olympic silver-medal marathoner Elana Meyer, and U.S. Olympic gold-medal cyclist Steve Hegg. The case of Australian modern pentathlete Alex Watson, who was sent home from the Seoul Olympics for registering a urinary caffeine level over the doping threshold, was highly publicized in Australia and continues to be discussed whenever the topic of caffeine in sport is raised. His case is such a compelling example of the difficulties associated with the position of caffeine on the list of banned substances that we have included an extended account of it in the appendix.

By 1999 there was a major change in the understanding of several issues related to caffeine use in sport. First, scientists and authorities were becoming aware of the limitations of urinary caffeine concentrations as a marker of caffeine use. As we discussed in chapter 2, urinary caffeine concentration reflects the small amount (~1%) of blood caffeine that escapes metabolism and is excreted unchanged. This clearance of caffeine varies widely among athletes and among occasions of use by the same athlete. On any given day for any given athlete, urinary caffeine levels could be influenced not only by the size of caffeine dose the athlete has taken but also by the clearance of caffeine into the urine and the amount of time that has elapsed between consuming the caffeine and producing the urine sample. Because these factors can vary greatly, it is easy to see that a one-off urine check isn't a consistent marker of how much caffeine an athlete has taken.

> I'm a regular coffee drinker. My usual is a cup of coffee in the morning and a cup in the afternoon if I have a hard workout. Despite my daily coffee use, I still feel I get a performance benefit from caffeine pills on race day. My races are usually pretty late—around 8 p.m.—so I have my morning coffee, an afternoon coffee 4 hours before race time, and then 150 mg (3 mg times my body mass) 1 hour before race time. It took me a couple years to figure out the right combination, but I feel like I've got it down to a science now that gives me the right focus and performance benefit without feeling too jittery.
>
> *Female Olympic 1,500-meter runner*

Second, as we showed in chapter 5, evidence was starting to accumulate from well-designed studies that performance benefits can be found with modest caffeine intakes (e.g., 2-3 mg/kg or 100-200 mg caffeine). Furthermore, caffeine works in a variety of intake protocols before and during exercise. Rather than being able to differentiate ergogenic uses of caffeine at high levels and social uses of caffeine, it was becoming clear that athletes could achieve performance benefits with caffeine intakes well within, or even below, the everyday caffeine use of the general population. Such intakes of caffeine are likely to be associated with low urinary caffeine levels, and in some cases, no detectable urinary caffeine.

## Evolution of Antidoping Rules (1999-2003)

The most important change in the landscape of caffeine and sport occurred as a result of changes in the methods and intentions of the major antidoping programs. The World Anti-Doping Agency (WADA) was created in 1999 as an independent international organization to promote, coordinate, and monitor the fight against doping in sport. It was set up with a unique model underpinned by the UNESCO International Convention against Doping in Sport, to which the governments of participating countries were signatories. It receives 50% of its funding from the Olympic Movement and 50% from governments. With a stated goal to "work towards a vision of the world where all athletes compete in a doping-free sporting environment" (www.wada-ama.org/), WADA's first job was to harmonize antidoping policies and rules among sporting organizations and governments around the world. On January 1, 2004, it took over the antidoping work of the IOC and instituted its first code and international standards.

A major change between the IOC antidoping program and the WADA program was the expansion of ways in which it detects and sanctions athletes who dope. Nonanalytical violations are now possible, which means athletes can be found guilty of a doping offense without the need for a positive urine or blood test. Other offenses include refusing to provide test samples as well as possessing, importing, or admitting the use of prohibited substances. The offenses can be noted from direct evidence as well as indirect evidence such as testimony of other people. Furthermore, people other than athletes can be found guilty of doping offenses, including manufacturers or agents who supply prohibited substances, doctors who administer or monitor these substances, and other support staff who enable doping practices.

I do not want my athletes using caffeine for training. I want them to be in tune with their bodies.

*Olympic sprint coach and Olympic gold medalist*

In the interim between forming WADA (1999) and implementing its work (2004), another code was put in place—the Olympic Movement Anti-Doping Code. This code included caffeine within the category of stimulants banned in competition, with an explanatory comment that for caffeine, the definition of a positive is a concentration in urine greater than 12 µg/ml (www.la84foundation .org/OlympicInformationCenter/OlympicReview/2000/OREXXVI32/ OREXXVI32zza.pdf). However, with the move toward nonanalytical positives, there were several interpretations of the wording of this code. It could have meant

- caffeine is permitted for competition use by athletes at doses that produce urinary caffeine concentrations below 12 µg/ml, or
- caffeine is a prohibited substance outright. Urinary caffeine concentrations >12 µg/ml are a reporting limit, but all observed or admitted uses of caffeine in competition constitute a doping offense.

These interpretations have widely differing and far-reaching outcomes. Indeed, discussions at a workshop on caffeine in sport held at the AIS in 2001 identified a range of issues related to the various positions that caffeine could have in the new antidoping code. These are summarized in table 7.1 and illustrate the considerable practical challenges of implementing the various ideas of where caffeine should sit in relation to antidoping. These challenges would require careful consideration in the implementation of the new antidoping code.

# WADA Code (2004)

On January 1, 2004, the World Anti-Doping Code came into effect in preparation for the Athens Olympic Games and remains the current standard. As a core component of WADA activities, it is supported by a comprehensive and far-reaching program of scientific research, education, testing, and detection of doping. The code is still based on a banned list, or more correctly, three lists of prohibited substances and methods that apply to in-competition situations, out-of-competition situations (i.e., all the time), and particular sports. A substance or method is included in the prohibited list if it satisfies any two of the following three criteria, all of which are weighted equally:

- It is performance enhancing.
- It represents an actual or potential health risk to an athlete.
- The use of the substance or method violates the spirit of sport.

**Table 7.1** Examples of Potential Rulings Regarding Caffeine Use in Sport

| Ruling | Underpinning rationale | Implications and issues |
| --- | --- | --- |
| Caffeine is a prohibited substance in competition in absolute terms (i.e., any amount). | • Caffeine is a stimulant; caffeine intake enhances sports performance.<br>• Caffeine is neither a nutrient nor a necessary part of the diet and athletes could be reasonably expected to remove it from their diets before competition. | • Athletes would not be able to consume any tea, coffee, cola drinks, chocolate, and so on in the period before and during competition.<br>• Strong educational messages would be needed to convey this message and its implications to sport.<br>• A limit of urinary caffeine content would need to be set at very low levels. Although some athletes would be able to consume caffeine and remain below this limit, a positive doping offense would also be deemed to occur if the athlete was observed or admitted to consuming a caffeine-containing product during the competition period.<br>• Presumably, the difficulty in removing all caffeine from the normal diet would result in a large number of positive doping offenses.<br>• Possession and trafficking issues would arise concerning the sale of tea, coffee, cola, and chocolate at sporting venues and the sponsorship of athletes, events, and sporting organizations by companies that manufacture these products. These activities would need to be banned to be consistent with the antidoping code.<br>• Even though caffeine intake is banned in competition, athletes would still be able to consume caffeine during training in a manner that benefits their performance and adaptation to the training program. |
| Caffeine is a prohibited substance only when consumed in competition settings in doses that produce urinary caffeine levels above a certain limit (to be determined). | A urinary caffeine limit should be set to discriminate between social and intentional use of caffeine, or at least to pick up only a few cases of very high caffeine use. | • It is impossible to find a limit that distinguishes between social and intentional use of caffeine. Caffeine intakes that enhance performance are indistinguishable from the caffeine intakes reported by the general population.<br>• Urinary caffeine levels vary among and within individuals, and there is no standardized collection of urine samples with regard to the timing between caffeine intake and sampling. Therefore, urinary caffeine limits do not treat caffeine use equally.<br>• Educational messages to athletes could contain information about levels of caffeine intake that are unlikely to produce a urinary caffeine level above the limit.<br>• Athletes should not investigate their urinary caffeine concentrations in relation to various levels of intake (trying to find how much caffeine they can take without producing a positive result for caffeine doping); this would be regarded as controlled doping.<br>• Issues related to possession and trafficking of caffeine (as outlined in ruling 1) may still apply. |

| Ruling | Underpinning rationale | Implications and issues |
|---|---|---|
| Caffeine is a prohibited substance only when intentionally consumed in competition settings in doses that produce urinary caffeine levels above a certain limit (to be determined). | A model similar to drunk-driving laws will prevent accidental cases of high caffeine levels. | As previously discussed, except for the following:<br>• Because urinary caffeine levels vary from person to person, and there is no standardized collection of urine samples with regard to the timing between caffeine intake and sampling, athletes should be allowed (or encouraged) to investigate what intakes of caffeine can be tolerated without producing a positive test, without any penalty or prejudice. The concept of controlled doping would not apply. |
| The prohibition on caffeine use in sport is removed. | • Caffeine is so entrenched in the normal diet that it is not practical to try to ban intake.<br>• There is no unfair advantage if the majority of athletes already consume caffeine and choose to consume it for social reasons.<br>• There are no health disadvantages to the intake of small amounts of caffeine.<br>• The ergogenic benefits of caffeine on performance, although worthwhile, are small. For example, they are similar in magnitude to the effects of consuming carbohydrate during an endurance event but less than the beneficial effects of consuming fluid to minimize dehydration. | • Offers a practical solution to a challenging situation.<br>• Avoids tainting common foods and drinks or common transactions in sport (e.g., sponsorship by companies that produce these products) with the odium of cheating.<br>• Research should target the smallest dose of caffeine that can produce an ergogenic benefit. Educational messages to athletes could promote the message that if they desire to use caffeine (socially or intentionally), small intakes of caffeine produce maximal effects. Athletes would be encouraged to reduce rather than increase their intakes of caffeine, thus minimizing the health implications and cost of using special products.<br>• The market for specialized sport products containing caffeine might increase, unless educational messages remove the perceived benefits of large doses of caffeine or the need for special food products. |

Adapted from L.M.Burke, 2001, Report from workshop on caffeine in sport, December 2001, Australian Institute of Sport, Canberra, Australia.

The list is compiled and reviewed annually by a WADA panel, following consultation with a wide group of sporting authorities and governments.

The initial and all subsequent updates of the WADA List of Prohibited Substances and Methods until the publication of this book (2013) have not included caffeine as a banned substance. This position allows athletes to consume caffeine either in their background diets or for the specific purpose of performance enhancement without fear of sanctions. The deliberations of WADA's List Expert Group and its exact reasons for deciding what substances are included on or excluded from the prohibited list are not accessible to the public, so we can't be aware of all the factors underpinning the decisions. However, the Questions and Answers section on WADA's website for both the 2011 and 2012 lists provide some of the rationale for its decision on caffeine (see table 7.2). The WADA list in 2013 did not include any special commentary related to caffeine, presumably because it felt the position on caffeine is now well understood.

**Table 7.2** Questions and Answers Provided by WADA to Accompany the Prohibited Lists in 2011 and 2012

| | 2011 | 2012 |
|---|---|---|
| What is the status of caffeine? | Caffeine was removed from the prohibited list in 2004. Its use in sport is not prohibited. | The status of caffeine has not changed from last year. Caffeine was removed from the prohibited list in 2004. Its use in sport is not prohibited. |
| | Arguments that led WADA to take caffeine off the list in 2004 include research indicating that caffeine can potentially decrease performance above the 12 µg/ml threshold that was historically used in sport. Many experts believe that caffeine is ubiquitous in beverages and food and that reducing the threshold might therefore create the risk of sanctioning athletes for social or diet consumption of caffeine. In addition, caffeine is metabolized at very different rates in individuals. | Many experts believe that caffeine is ubiquitous in beverages and food and that reducing the threshold might therefore create the risk of sanctioning athletes for social or diet consumption of caffeine. In addition, caffeine is metabolized at very different rates in individuals. |
| | Caffeine is part of WADA's Monitoring Program. This program includes substances that are not prohibited in sport but that WADA monitors in order to detect patterns of misuse. The 2010 Monitoring Program did not reveal global patterns of caffeine misuse in sport. Caffeine will remain part of the Monitoring Program in 2011. | Caffeine is part of WADA's Monitoring Program. This program includes substances that are not prohibited in sport but that WADA monitors in order to detect patterns of misuse. The 2010 and 2011 Monitoring Programs did not reveal specific global patterns of caffeine misuse in sport, although a significant increase in consumption in the athletic population is observed. |

Adapted, by permission, from (1) World Anti-Doping Agency, 2010, Questions and answers on 2011 prohibited list. [Online]. Available: www.wada-ama.org/en/Resources/Q-and-A/2011-Prohibited-List/ [October 20, 2011] and (2) World Anti-Doping Agency, 2011, Questions and answers on 2012 prohibited list. [Online]. Available: www.wada-ama.org/en/Resources/Q-and-A/2012-Prohibited-List/ [March 1, 2013].

It should be noted, however, that caffeine is still on the list of banned drug classes of the NCAA, the body governing college sport in the United States. A doping infringement is cited if urinary caffeine concentrations exceed 15 µg/ml.

Caffeine remains on the WADA Monitoring Program, meaning that caffeine concentrations are still measured in urine samples collected by in-competition antidoping monitoring as a means of detecting patterns of misuse in sport. This has allowed some examination of the impact of removing caffeine from the prohibited list. As seen in chapter 4, some studies have found a high prevalence of caffeine use for perceived ergogenic effects from the self-reported practices of select groups of athletes.

However, measurement of more than 4,600 urine samples collected across 56 sports by an accredited Belgian laboratory in 2004 found no increase in mean urinary caffeine concentrations compared with results from 1993 to 2002 (see chapter 4 for more details). The mean caffeine concentration in samples in 2004 was 1.12 µg/ml, in comparison to a finding of 1.22 µg/ml from more than 11,000 samples collected in the earlier period. The 2004 study noted differences in caffeine use between sports, with an increased average concentration and a larger percentage of higher urinary caffeine concentrations (defined as >4 µg/ml) in cycling and strength and power sports compared with other sports. Cycling showed an apparent increase in the percentage of higher urinary caffeine concentrations in 2004, whereas there was a decrease in this outcome in swimming and basketball. Overall there was a decrease in the percentage of urine samples showing caffeine concentrations below the detectable range, and there was no increase in the percentage of samples with a concentration above 12 µg/ml. Only six samples had a concentration above the former cutoff level.

An even larger study from a doping-control laboratory in Madrid reported on their measures of urinary caffeine from more than 20,000 samples collected across sporting events from 2004 to 2008. Again, they found no increase in mean urinary caffeine concentrations across these years and found a similarly low number of samples above the old doping threshold (see chapter 4 for details). The authors tried to explain why there appear to be no changes in the patterns of caffeine use over the past decade due to the changes in caffeine's status in antidoping programs. They speculated that during the time when caffeine was included on IOC and WADA prohibited lists (1984-2004), competitors benefited from taking low to moderate caffeine doses (3-6 mg/kg) and avoided doses that they thought would exceed the urine caffeine threshold deemed as a doping offense. However, the removal of caffeine from the prohibited list in 2004 coincided with newer information showing that higher doses of caffeine do not achieve better performance outcomes and are therefore unnecessary (see chapter 5).

When I first started taking caffeine for competition, I was not a coffee drinker, and it had a huge effect on me. I used to take a 100 mg pill 60 minutes before the start of the race, but I got too tense and I felt that it had a negative effect on my swim performance because my muscles were too tight. Because of that, I now take the same amount at the beginning of the bike leg to get a performance boost toward the end of the race.

*Female triathlete, three-time Olympian, European Championship silver medalist*

Continued monitoring needs to take place—and be published—before firm conclusions can be made about the long-term effect of removing caffeine from the list of prohibited substances. Similarly, despite the limitations of urinary caffeine concentrations as a reflection of caffeine use, monitoring will be valuable to investigate apparent changes in the culture and practice of caffeine use among athletes. Nevertheless there seems to be little evidence of systematic increases in the use or misuse of caffeine at the highest levels of sport. Information on the WADA website in relation to caffeine states that the results of the 2010 monitoring program did not show cause for concern regarding changes in caffeine use. Notes on the 2011 program state that it observed a "significant increase in (caffeine) consumption in the athletic population" (www.wada-ama. org/en/Science-Medicine/Prohibited-List/QA-on-2012-Prohibited-List.), without providing information on whether this meant more athletes were recording detectable levels of caffeine in their urine or whether these urinary caffeine levels had increased compared with previous years. Nevertheless, the current WADA position is that it has not detected global patterns of caffeine misuse.

## Not the End of the Story

In 2004, many people, including these authors, thought the story of caffeine in sport might end happily ever after. The concluding chapter might have gone something like this:

- New research shows that low to moderate doses of caffeine, consistent with safe and healthy levels of caffeine intake in the normal population, can enhance sports performance. The message spreads that there is no additional benefit from larger caffeine doses.

- The main antidoping agency provides unambiguous advice that athletes may take caffeine in relation to competition, either for performance-enhancing purposes or as part of their everyday diet. The decision is based on this emerging knowledge and a pragmatic approach to the difficulties of prohibiting low levels of a product that is ingrained in our dietary behaviors and social practices.

- Sport scientists are provided with a greater ability to undertake transparent research programs and education activities to make coaches and athletes better aware of the benefits and disadvantages of caffeine use in sport. Knowledge accumulates to promote a more targeted and effective use of caffeine.

- Greater dissemination of this emerging information that the benefits of caffeine occur at small to moderate doses, and of the presence of individual variability and potential side effects in response to caffeine intake, leads to a reduction in total caffeine use and caffeine misuse by athletes.

- Our understanding of the role of caffeine in sports performance has approached a full circle. After decades of believing that caffeine offered a benefit to sports performance only when used in specific large doses and protocols, it now appears that patterns mimicking the everyday use of caffeine to enhance well-being and the performance of daily activities also apply to sport.

However, real life has produced a more complicated outcome, and at the time of writing this book, it appears that the end is still not in sight.

Since the removal of caffeine from the WADA List of Prohibited Substances and Methods in 2004, controversial events regarding caffeine supplementation by athletes have surfaced, showcasing problems that are entrenched and complex. Episodes that have exposed caffeine practices by athletes have resulted in intense media scrutiny, public outcry, and debates among sports medicine professionals, antidoping personnel, sport authorities, and athletes. Several of these controversies are illuminated in the sidebars in this chapter and in chapter 8.

At the heart of these episodes are situations of caffeine abuse by some athletes. Testimonials by athletes have revealed caffeine doses that are excessive both in terms of normal daily caffeine use and the new evidence of the threshold of benefits from caffeine intake at about 3 mg/kg. In addition, there have been admissions of the use of sleeping tablets to combat the poor sleep associated with caffeine use during competition. Other caffeine controversies in sport have included its combination with other stimulants, such as pseudoephedrine, ephedrine, and methylhexaneamine, in the quest for an additional performance boost. (This situation is typically seen with recreational athletes or athletes who participate in sports without antidoping codes, since these other stimulants are banned under the WADA code.) A final controversy involves the use of caffeine by young athletes.

# Anatomy of a Caffeine Controversy, Part 1

In 2005, caffeine use in sport hit the frontlines of the Australian sporting media following a television show where professional Australian rules football players described match-day strategies, which included taking caffeine tablets. Many media reports followed in which athletes from a range of sports and sporting codes were asked about their own competition habits with caffeine. It was a story that wouldn't go away.

Many of the well-known football stars and other athletes made candid and public statements about their use of caffeine, often in the form of caffeine tablets and usually taken before competitive events. Some of these have been provided in the Athlete Caffeine Experience comments throughout this book. The statements included information that caffeine was scientifically proven to enhance the performance of their specific sports and that caffeine was not a banned substance within the antidoping codes of their sports. Some players also noted that their caffeine use was monitored by club fitness and medical staff and that they were fully aware of both the benefits and side effects of caffeine.

However, many high-profile coaches, sports medicine professionals, and sport administrators spoke out in disagreement with the views and practices of these athletes. Comments on television programs, on radio shows, and in the written press included the view that such admissions are not suitable from role models for junior sportspeople:

**Rodney Eade, Australian rules football coach (Western Bulldogs):** "I think it's probably irresponsible for players and coaches to talk about tablets openly. It just sends the wrong message."

**Terry Wallace, coach (Richmond Tigers):** "If I thought that we were responsible for 15- and 16-year-old kids sneaking down to the local store to pick up NoDoz because they thought that was going to make the difference between them making the Northern Knights or the Collaroy Cannons, I'd be shattered."

Some prominent physicians declared the practices to have medical risk:

**Dr. Peter Larkins, sports physician:** "I think that the comments by George Gregan and other high-profile athletes are most unhealthy. . . .You're talking about overstimulation. You're talking about increase in your heart rate, you're talking about a tremor, you're talking about increases and changes in fine motor control or technique because you might be overaroused and anxious and irritable, even."

It was alleged that caffeine use by athletes has dramatically increased:

**Dr. Peter Larkins:** "Removing caffeine from the banned list has resulted in an increased explosion of use of caffeine in sport."

Finally, there was discussion that caffeine use by athletes, despite its removal from the list of prohibited substances, was unethical:

**David Howman, WADA:** "This is, I suppose, bordering on cheating. If it's not on the list it's not cheating but it's bordering, and it's saying 'well let's take every step now,' each sport's got to be in a position whether it determines that's acceptable for it or not. I think society's got to make that same sort of decision."

Other statements from WADA added confusion by suggesting that caffeine was previously unknown as an enhancer of sports performance and that it would be reconsidered for a return to the prohibited list:

**Dick Pound, WADA chairman:** "The interesting thing in this debate is not that a lot of Australian players and athletes have come out saying that they have taken caffeine, but that the AIS says it is performance enhancing with research backing up their claims and recommending how it should be taken. Having heard this, our list committee will take another look at it."

The controversy continued with much media scrutiny for months.

Sources: M. Fuller, 2005, "Gregan admits taking pre-game caffeine dose," *The Age*, Melbourne, Australia: May 18, 2005. [Online]. Available: www.theage.com.au/news/Union/Gregan-admits-taking-pregame-caffeine-dose/2005/05/17/1116095965523.html [March 4, 2013]; J. Magney, 2005, "Agency may ban caffeine again," *The Age*, Melbourne, Australia: May 19, 2005. [Online]. Available: www.theage.com.au/news/Sport/Agency-may-ban-caffeine-again/2005/05/18/1116361614219.html [March 4, 2013]; TV program transcript, Australian Broadcasting Corporation, May 18, 2005. [Online]. Available: www.abc.net.au/7.30/content/2005/s1371799.htm [March 4, 2013].

None of these situations is condoned by the authors of this book. In fact, none is a useful or necessary part of caffeine use in sport. Many sport scientists, sports medicine professionals, and sport authorities have spoken up during such public controversies, hoping to use the opportunity to educate athletes about more appropriate ways to use caffeine in sport. Many hope that such publicity will allow athletes to hear about new research concerning caffeine and updates on best practice for caffeine use. However, the typical result is outcry from their peers and from the public, which continues to fuel the debate, often adding misinformation and emotion rather than clarity or calm to the discussion. Although the specific incident gradually disappears from discussion, the tension regarding caffeine use by athletes remains.

**Table 7.3**  Emotive Areas of Belief Regarding Caffeine

| Perception | Reality | Context |
|---|---|---|
| Some sources of caffeine (particularly caffeine pills) are inherently worse than others even if the dose is identical. | All sources of caffeine are chemically identical and achieve the same effects on the body. In fact, some of the caffeine sources with a poor reputation have the advantage of providing a known amount of caffeine; many socially acceptable caffeine sources (e.g., coffee) can provide unknown and potentially larger caffeine doses. | Similar irrational views exist outside the sporting context: The use of caffeine pills by truck drivers to assist alertness while driving is considered bad while driver-alert programs that sponsor coffee stations at roadside locations are providing a valuable service. Within the military, use of caffeine aids (gums and pills) to combat battle fatigue is considered lifesaving. |
| Caffeine use by athletes contravenes fair play or the ethics of sport. | Although athletes can have their own set of ethics and morals, the bigger framework involves an externally determined set of strict codes and rules of conduct. Caffeine is a permitted substance within the WADA code, and the ethics of sport is one of the three factors that were considered in the decision-making process. | Many people disagree with the offside rule in soccer. However, soccer is played according to the FIFA code rather than personal views on the sense and value of individual rules. |
| Caffeine is a stimulant that allows athletes to achieve a superhuman advantage. | Caffeine exerts its major effect by reducing the perception or demonstration of fatigue that occurs when an activity is undertaken for a prolonged time. It works by allowing people to work at their normal or optimal level for longer. The benefit to performance is typically within the range of a 1% to 3% improvement, which is substantial to the outcomes of high-level sport. This benefit is of a similar magnitude, however, to the effects of consuming carbohydrate during sports longer than 60 min or of drinking fluid to reduce dehydration. | Most people use caffeine in their everyday lives to enhance their well-being and alertness and to reduce the fatigue that manifests while undertaking occupational or recreational activities. |
| Athletes use much larger doses of caffeine than normal dietary intakes, and antidoping agencies are concerned that caffeine use has dramatically increased since caffeine was removed from the banned list. | Doses of caffeine associated with performance enhancement are similar to normal dietary intakes by adults in the general population. Monitoring programs have failed to find evidence of a widespread or increasing prevalence of supplemental practices by athletes involving very large amounts of caffeine. | Some sedentary people abuse caffeine—consuming it in excessive quantities, at inappropriate times, or in conjunction with alcohol or other stimulants. All situations of poor caffeine use should be addressed. |

| Perception | Reality | Context |
|---|---|---|
| Sport science and sports medicine professionals shouldn't be encouraging athletes to take caffeine. | Many athletes are already using caffeine related to sports performance but in ways that don't represent best practice—most often, in doses that are much larger than needed and inappropriate at times. The experience of many sport science and sports medicine professionals is that engaging with athletes to develop individualized caffeine use protocols often leads to a reduced caffeine intake—low doses used on fewer occasions and reduced social caffeine intake so that caffeine intake is targeted to training and competition performance. | Sport science and sports medicine professionals work with athletes to achieve performance enhancement from a large number of techniques that are safe, effective, and legal. |
| Elite athletes are role models to young athletes and shouldn't be sending a message that caffeine use is a required part of sports performance. | Messages to young people regarding sports performance should promote the need for a strong base built on maturation in age and experience in a sport and the big picture of healthy eating, recovery strategies, good equipment, and coaching. Strategies such as caffeine supplementation have a role as sprinkles on the icing on the cake. | Many of the training and competition strategies undertaken by elite athletes are not suitable for young athletes—for example, the number of hours spent in training, the size of the weights lifted in a gym workout, and the money spent on equipment. |

At least part of the problem is that many people have strong and often irrational beliefs about caffeine that cloud their judgment and ability to see other viewpoints. Table 7.3 summarizes some of these ideas, trying to provide a more logical and evidence-based discussion of the issues. Currently, there is a gulf between the scientific evidence regarding safe and effective use of caffeine in sport, the practices of some athletes, and the beliefs of some members of the public. Finding the balance will require reeducation and some concessions from everyone involved.

# The Bottom Line

Caffeine was removed from the prohibited list of the WADA code on January 1, 2004, and its use in sport is not prohibited. The rationale for this change includes recognition that caffeine enhances performance at doses that are indistinguishable from social caffeine use, and that the previous practice of monitoring caffeine use via urinary caffeine concentrations is not reliable. Caffeine is part of WADA's Monitoring Program, which monitors substances to detect patterns of misuse in sport. This program has not revealed global patterns of misuse of caffeine in sport.

Nevertheless, there is evidence that some athletes do not follow best practice or evidence-based protocols for caffeine use in training, competition performance, or social intake of caffeine. Developing programs to combat real or perceived misuse of caffeine in sport is challenged by several factors, including a lack of up-to-date knowledge by athletes, coaches, and even sports medicine practitioners regarding caffeine and sports performance. Community members are rightly concerned about caffeine misuse in sport. However, they often also hold emotional views about caffeine that are neither factual nor rational. These views exacerbate the perception of the extent and nature of true problems.

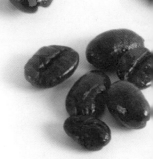

# Chapter

# 8

# Recovery and Other Considerations

Back in the good old days, athletes just used to worry about the day of the game or race. Get to the starting line or starting siren. Go hard. Go home. Life was simple.

The modern world of sport science, however, has a far more sophisticated approach to managing performance goals. We now recognize the benefits of periodized training and the importance of recovery and adaptation between sessions. We also realize that the gold medal or championship trophy is often awarded after a series of games or heats and finals. In other words, we need to think from day to day and join the dots between workouts or competition. Recovery is now an industry.

With that in mind, there are some additional issues that athletes need to consider in relation to caffeine and performance. We will file them under the category of recovery, but they may also flow into other areas of everyday life or performance.

## Hydration

We all know that caffeine is a diuretic. A cup of coffee makes us dash to the restroom and for every cup we drink, we need to add another glass of water to our daily eight. That can't be good for athletes who are already losing buckets of sweat during exercise, right? Or for the plane flight home after the race? After all, the airline magazine on your flight home carries a warning along the lines of "drink tea and coffee in moderation since these are diuretics and will increase

> It isn't for us to decide what we can and can't take: the world anti-doping authorities make those decisions and we abide by them. I appreciate these rules, and have no wish to see them relax, as I never want to see the day when competitors in any sport are sacrificing their health in pursuit of greatness. But if there is something out there that is legal, won't hurt you and will give you an edge, I think an athlete would be mad to ignore it. Yet, that was what some commentators and doctors' groups wanted me to do in May 2005, after it was revealed that I was taking caffeine tablets to assist my performance.
>
> *George Gregan (2009, p. 250)*

your dehydration," so it must be serious. Drinking caffeinated drinks before and during exercise on a hot day is particularly risky because your performance will go down the toilet. The threat to hydration or rehydration probably rates as one of the best known facts about caffeine.

Except that it's not true. Several experts have recently tried to debunk this old wives' tale about caffeine and dehydration. We like the work of Professor Lawrence Armstrong because it takes into account issues related to exercise. Here are some of his observations from 2002 and 2005.

- A diuretic is a substance that increases the production of urine. By definition, water or any drink consumed in large volumes is a diuretic. The effect of any fluid on body hydration is judged by the balance sheet of how much the body retains of any volume that is consumed.

- Caffeine is a weak diuretic. It may influence the volume of urine production and loss by acting on some of the hormones involved in urine production, and it may also influence the loss of electrolytes in urine. However, tolerance to the diuretic effects of caffeine is acquired in as little as 4 or 5 days of regular caffeine intake. Studies in the 1920s showed that for someone who hadn't consumed caffeine in more than 60 days, a dose as little as 0.5 g/kg (e.g., 35 mg for a 70 kg person) caused a noticeable increase in urine losses. However, regular caffeine intake created a tolerance to the diuretic effect such that a dose of 1.12 g/kg was needed before an effect on urine losses was detectable.

- A variety of studies have compared urine losses when subjects consumed caffeine with or as part of a beverage compared with water or a noncaffeinated control or placebo condition. Most were undertaken in sedentary conditions, and a couple were undertaken after exercise or during exercise. Caffeine doses ranged from low (~100 mg) to high (~700 mg) and urine losses were tracked for several hours (up to 24 hours). In some cases, the differences in urine losses between caffeine and no caffeine were judged to be similar; in others, the urine losses in the caffeine trial were significantly greater according to a statistical interpretation. Small to moderate intakes of caffeine (<250 mg) were found to have minimal effects on urine losses, and the mean effect of caffeine ranged from actually reducing urine losses to increasing urine losses by 50 to 100 ml. Importantly, in all situations, the majority of the drink volume consumed with caffeine was retained, so the subjects gained fluid over the course of the trial.

- When healthy people were followed over 11 days in which their caffeine intake was first stabilized for 6 days and then manipulated for 5 days at zero, low (3 mg/kg), or moderate (6 mg/kg) levels, there was no significant effect on urine production or characteristics.

Armstrong concluded that the consumption of caffeine doesn't pose a threat to hydration levels via its alleged diuretic actions, particularly in small to moderate doses, and that any effects on urine losses are small and unimportant. A systematic review by Professor Ron Maughan, who we introduced in the preface of this book, came to a similar conclusion (Maughan and Griffin 2003). The summary to this publication stated that

> the available literature suggests that acute ingestion of caffeine in large doses (at least 250-300 mg) . . . results in a short-term stimulation of urine output in individuals who have been deprived of caffeine for a period of days or weeks. A profound tolerance to the diuretic and other effects of caffeine develops, however, and the actions are much diminished in individuals who regularly consume tea or coffee. Doses of caffeine equivalent to the amount normally found in standard servings of tea, coffee and carbonated soft drinks appear to have no diuretic action. . . . The most ecologically valid of the published studies offers no support for the suggestion that consumption of caffeine-containing beverages as part of a normal lifestyle leads to fluid loss in excess of the volume ingested or is associated with poor hydration status. Therefore, there would appear to be no clear basis for refraining from caffeine-containing drinks in situations where fluid balance might be compromised.

Before leaving the issue of caffeine and hydration, we should examine two specific variations on this theme. Urine losses contribute to fluid balance, of course, but the big picture is far more complicated than that. The minus side of fluid balance also includes sweat losses, and it has been proposed that caffeine intake might increase sweat rates either by directly affecting the sweat glands or by raising metabolic rate and body temperature. This might be of greatest importance to consider when an athlete is exercising in hot weather, and caffeine use might have an effect on heat regulation as well as hydration. Several studies have examined this issue, and in addition to measuring the individual components of fluid balance, they have looked at the bottom line of total fluid balance, body temperature regulation, and performance. The findings have been consistent: Caffeine intake before and during exercise has zero to minor effect on sweat losses, body temperature, and urine losses during exercise. However, there is no detriment to total hydration, temperature control, or performance compared with trials without caffeine. Therefore, decisions to use moderate doses of caffeine before and during exercise in hot conditions need not be overly concerned about heat and hydration.

The final issue that we need to address regarding caffeine and hydration is the plus side of the fluid balance sheet. A key consideration in real life is that a drink needs to be consumed before it contributes to body fluid levels. As much as thirst is important, people also drink according to habit, social behavior, fluid availability and personal preferences. As we have seen in chapter 4, caffeine-containing drinks score highly in each of these areas. Beverages such as tea, coffee, cola drinks, and in some populations, energy drinks, contribute a significant volume of our daily voluntary intake of fluid. In some cases, there may be good reasons to suggest we should reduce our total or specific intake of these drinks. We now know that fluid balance isn't likely to be one of these reasons, although we know of people who swear that they have to get up in the night to go to the bathroom if they drink caffeine-containing drinks before bed. But, we also need to recognize the value of the fluid that they do contribute to our daily balance. If people were to suddenly give up their normal intake of caffeinated beverages, the net effect might be a reduction in fluid intake until they found other drinks that were similarly enjoyable, ubiquitous, and easy to ingrain into their habits and social routines. The Perfect Study sidebar illustrates a case in point.

## Refueling

A workout or competitive event of sufficient intensity and length can deplete or at least substantially reduce the muscle stores of glycogen. Replacing these fuel stores is a priority in many recovery situations, notably where there is a short time until the next important training session or event. The key nutrient is carbohydrate, and there are well-established guidelines regarding the timing and amount of carbohydrate that should be consumed to restore muscle glycogen content. In some situations, athletes might benefit from tactics that increase muscle glycogen storage rates in general or from a given amount of dietary carbohydrate. By the same token, a factor that reduces muscle glycogen storage from a carbohydrate meal would be considered counterproductive.

# The Perfect Study

So, the in-flight magazine tells you that tea, coffee, and cola are diuretics and should be consumed in moderation during the flight due to their ability to dehydrate you. Unfortunately, when the meal service or snack tray comes around, the flight attendants offer you cups of the stuff. What should you do? Avoid the poisoned chalice, or do what you do every other day of your life and drink them? Just how dehydrated will you become? Being intrepid scientists, we love the idea of a challenge. Here's the study we would like to do.

On several long-haul flights, we would divide the plane down the middle. Passengers on one side would be told to take heed of in-flight directions and avoid all tea, coffee, and cola drinks. The other passengers would be instructed to take a walk on the wild side and drink whatever they feel like and normally do. Which group do you predict would be better hydrated at the end of the flight?

We feel pretty sure that the wild-side passengers would come out on top. Would we bet our PhDs on the outcome? Probably. The reason we feel so cocky is because we know that hydration levels are a balance between intake (the volume of fluid that a person drinks) and output (the amount that goes down the toilet). Although the focus with caffeine-containing drinks has been on the output side—and we now know that this is overstated—we recognize that these drinks contribute a significant source of fluid to the plus side of the balance sheet. So, what happens when people are suddenly prevented from drinking beverages that are enjoyable, accessible, and part of their daily behavior? We predict that a significantly smaller volume of fluid would be consumed because

- people will not drink as much of an alternative beverage choice that they don't really like, and some may even decline to take a drink at all, and
- if the only accessible choices are not suitable (i.e., the tea and coffee service), no fluid will be consumed and there may not be other opportunities to make up for this.

Therefore, we think that the major effect on hydration would come from a failure to compensate for habitual drinking practices, making the traditional advice on caffeinated drinks needless and potentially negative. This doesn't mean that passengers should take a free-for-all approach to caffeine during long flights; in fact, we advise them to consider their intake of caffeine-containing drinks in view of the sleep patterns they need to adjust to in the time zone of their destination. We just don't think that the advice on dehydrating drinks stacks up.

We are ready to go, should an airline like to support such a research project. The final condition is that we think it would be best tested on economy passengers who are a more captive audience in terms of in-flight hospitality and their ability to move around the craft to look after their own needs. Of course, as researchers we would need to remove ourselves from the immediate environment so that we don't influence people's behavior and contaminate the data. The best option would be for us to observe from the distance of first class. Science is often a tough business.

Circumstantial evidence has suggested both a positive and negative role for caffeine in relation to postexercise refueling. Sedentary people who undertake an OGTT—an investigation of how the body handles the consumption of a substantial glucose dose (~1 g/kg) after an overnight fast—generally show a reduced ability to lower their blood sugar levels if they have been given a dose of caffeine beforehand. The OGTT is used to indicate the presence or risk of diabetes and is a measure of how well a person's muscles can take up and store glucose. The observed effect of caffeine on the OGTT might suggest that it impairs muscle glycogen synthesis. On the other hand, several studies of carbohydrate intake during exercise in trained people have shown that caffeine increases the use of this carbohydrate as a muscle fuel. This suggests improved uptake of glucose into the muscle following caffeine intake.

Studies that have specifically investigated the effect of caffeine on glycogen storage during recovery after exercise have shown mixed results. Early work found no impairment of glycogen resynthesis after prolonged exercise when a caffeine intake equal to 6 mg/kg was consumed before and during exercise in conjunction with postexercise carbohydrate intake. However, David Pedersen and our colleagues (2008) at RMIT University in Melbourne received much publicity when they reported the highest rates of muscle glycogen storage ever measured in the recovery from exhaustive exercise. The strategy that achieved this feat during the 4-hour refueling period involved high levels of caffeine (a total of 8 mg/kg) added to high rates of carbohydrate intake (a total of 4 g/kg). The caffeine dose increased glycogen storage by 66% compared with a trial using carbohydrate intake alone, with the advantage seeming to relate to higher blood concentrations of glucose and insulin associated with caffeine intake.

5-Hour Energy got plenty of TV time Sunday during the final round of the 112th U.S. Open. Just not exactly in the set of circumstances it might have preferred. The energy drink . . . is the chief sponsor of golfer Jim Furyk, who led the Open going into Sunday before a stunning collapse over the final few holes. His collapse led to a stream of jokes in news stories and online. "5-Hour Energy to come out with new product with Furyk on it: 3 Hour & 46 Minute Energy," CNBC sports reporter Darren Rovell tweeted Sunday.

*Bill Shea (2012)*

Other researchers from Liverpool John Moores University followed up the practicality of this finding by having athletes repeat a trial in which they did two fuel-demanding exercise sessions in the same day. The first session depleted muscle glycogen stores and was followed 4 hours later by a high-intensity interval test to fatigue known as the Loughborough Intermittent Shuttle Test (LIST). Between each session athletes received a carbohydrate-rich drink providing an hourly dose equal to 1.2 g/kg. In one trial, the drink also contained caffeine adding up to a total dose of 8 mg/kg, as used in the RMIT study. Exercise capacity during the LIST was significantly longer in the carbohydrate and caffeine trial (~48 min) than with carbohydrate alone (~32 minutes). Although glycogen stores weren't measured in this study, the researchers suggested that the enhanced endurance in the second exercise task may have been due to better refueling after the first exercise bout. Of course, the improvement may have simply been a direct result of the effect of prior caffeine intake on exercise, as we explored in chapter 5.

More recently, however, a 2012 study from Professor Luc van Loon's lab in the Netherlands, led by colleague Milou Beelen, reexamined this caffeine and glycogen storage issue and was not able to corroborate the findings. They exercised trained cyclists to deplete glycogen in the morning on two occasions, followed by a 6 h recovery period where subjects ingested high amounts of carbohydrate (1.2 g/kg per hour) with or without high doses of caffeine (1.7 g/kg per hour for a total >8 mg/kg). The carbohydrate and caffeine were given every 30 min during recovery, and high plasma caffeine levels were reached. The glycogen resynthesis rates were identical with or without caffeine, even when individual types of muscle fiber were examined separately. The glucose absorption from the gut and overall plasma glucose concentrations also were not different. It is not clear why these results contradict the findings of the RMIT University research since the studies both used trained subjects and high levels of carbohydrate and caffeine.

> It was about 2:30 a.m. by the time we won the third set. Mike was drinking Coke during the match, and basically you keep yourself going on sugar and caffeine. They keep you amped up for hours so it can be really hard to get to sleep.
>
> *U.S. professional tennis players Rob and Mike Bryan (2012)*

Before any more work is undertaken on this topic, it should be noted that large amounts of caffeine are apparently needed to have an effect on glycogen storage. As we will find in the final part of this chapter, the effects of caffeine on sleep are of major importance. Therefore, when overnight refueling is the question at hand, it may be counterproductive to use caffeine to promote muscle fuel recovery at the expense of restful sleep.

## Postexercise Soreness

In chapter 2, we noted that caffeine has mild analgesic effects that block the perception of pain during exercise. This may sometimes contribute to the ability of caffeine to enhance sports performance or to allow the athlete to train harder.

This effect may also be useful after exercise to mask the pain associated with the DOMS (delayed-onset muscle soreness) that occurs in the days after unaccustomed exercise, particularly after eccentric exercise. Some studies in humans and rats have found that caffeine can reduce inflammation following damaging exercise or reduce the discomfort of DOMS. It is difficult to know how important these effects are or whether these findings could lead to specific recommendations to consume caffeine in the aftermath of exercise. At the moment, it is best to consider them as a valuable side effect of a preexisting caffeine habit. In addition, it explains why it is often possible to buy over-the-counter painkillers such as Excedrin that contain a small amount of caffeine (e.g., 65 mg) in addition to the traditional compounds such as aspirin or acetaminophen.

## Immune System

Exercise is generally regarded as a healthy activity that strengthens the immune system. However, and although there is some debate about this, there is reasonable evidence that heavy exercise actually suppresses the immune system, making athletes more susceptible to upper-respiratory tract infections (colds) after single bouts of prolonged exhaustive exercise, during periods of intensive training, and around the time of competition. Being sick has a major impact on performance if it stops the athlete from training consistently or if it coincides with a major event.

It is difficult to investigate the immune system and illness. The immune system depends on a huge number of intercommunicating cells and chemicals, many of which can be studied individually without knowing how they will affect how often or when a person will succumb to an infection. Tracking illness itself is equally tricky because it is hard to come up with a universal code to record the presence and severity of symptoms. More importantly, because most people don't get sick that often, you need studies involving large numbers of people or long periods of investigation before you can see if any intervention changes patterns of illness. Rest assured, however, that experts in sports medicine and science are busily trying to understand the relationship between exercise and the immune system and how to stop athletes from becoming sick too often or at the worst times.

Caffeine has cropped up among the array of factors that seem to alter the activity of immune cells, and, funnily enough, in a good way. Several studies have shown that both low and moderate doses of caffeine can stimulate the activity of natural killer (NK) cells via an adenosine-mediated effect after a 1-hour bout of high-intensity exercise. We are in the early days of researching the immune system, and we have no idea how this integrates into the overall immune system activity or the functional endpoint of getting sick. Watch this area for future results.

# Physique Changes

Because caffeine increases metabolic rate slightly, it has been proposed that it might increase daily energy expenditure and assist in weight control or weight loss. This explains the inclusion of caffeine in some popular weight-loss supplements, the so-called thermogenics, along with other stimulant ingredients. There isn't a great amount of evidence to support the use of low to moderate amounts of caffeine alone for weight loss. In these doses, the effects are probably too small to be significant. For example, a study of college students who undertook an 8-week training program, combined with a daily supplement providing either 200 mg of caffeine or a placebo, found no difference in the changes in fitness levels or body composition changes between groups.

> American sprinter Inger Miller, world champion at 200 meters, was stripped of her bronze medal at the 1999 world indoor championships in Japan when she tested positive for caffeine.

The use of large caffeine doses or combinations with other stimulants starts to move into the territory where side effects and health effects are more important than any effect on body fat. There is some evidence that caffeine combined with green tea extract can increase fat oxidation and metabolic rate. It probably only accounts for a small amount of fat loss above what can be achieved by an energy-controlled approach to diet and exercise. The bottom line, however, is that because the regulation of fat-loss supplements is often limited or unenforced, we don't recommend them. And if you are thinking that your normal caffeine intake might help to burn excess calories, be warned that the sugar content of energy drinks or the cream in the giant frappé far exceed the capacity of caffeine to increase metabolic rate.

# Sleep

Caffeine has a profound effect on sleep, reducing total sleep time, increasing the time taken to fall asleep, and changing the quality of sleep by reducing the amount of time spent in deep sleep. The effects of caffeine on sleep are related to the size of the dose, the level of tolerance to caffeine that can be developed, and individual differences among people. Because sleep plays an important role in recovery between exercise sessions, there is a fine line between enjoying the benefits of caffeine for performance or lifestyle and sacrificing the benefits of sleep. Many of us do a tango around this fine line in our everyday lives. Getting the balance wrong during training could lead to poor sleep followed by ineffective workouts the next day. Or, it can lead to scrambling with more caffeine the next day to rescue the situation, which then often spirals into the vicious caffeine cycle.

The competition scenario can be even trickier to get right. Several other characteristics are added to the mix when it comes to competition (note that these characteristics also exist in the training scenario for some people):

- The atmosphere, expectancy, and exercise intensity of competition lead to a heightened level of arousal in the athlete from which it can be difficult to fall asleep.

- In some sports, the outcome of the event requires a series of bouts, races, or matches that are spread over several days. The accumulation of poor recovery between sessions can add to the accumulation of fatigue from all-out efforts just when performance is becoming crucial.

- In some sports, competition finishes late at night. There may already be a short turnaround to the next day's timetable, which needs to include drug testing, media interviews, debriefs, equipment management, travel, eating, and more. The time for sleep is already short and the athlete needs to make the most of it.

- Some competitions involve travel to new locations with new sleeping arrangements (a new bed, an unaccustomed roommate, a noisy environment). This alters accustomed sleep hygiene patterns and creates challenges to restful sleep.

Most of us have stories about the effect of caffeine on our sleep habits. However, studying sleep in a laboratory is a science that uses polysomnography to monitor body functions, including brain waves, eye movements, muscle activity, skeletal muscle activation, and heart rhythm. Other devices, such as sleep actigraphs, can be worn as wristwatches to monitor sleep and sleepiness over the whole day in the athlete's own environment and everyday life.

Sleep involves a series of cycles, each lasting about 90 to 110 minutes, that move through various stages associated with specific brain activities. The usual pattern is as follows:

- Stage 1 sleep: Light sleep during which it is easy to wake up. You may experience a drifting in and out of sleep, a feeling that you haven't been to sleep, and sudden muscle jerks or hallucinogenic episodes such as hearing your name.

- Stage 2 sleep: Takes up about 50% of the cycle. Eye movement stops and brain waves become slower, with brief bursts of rapid brain activity.

- Stage 3 sleep: First stage of deep sleep with a combination of slow brain waves and some faster waves. It can be difficult to wake up from this sleep, and if you do, you may feel groggy and disorientated.

- Stage 4 sleep: Second stage of deep sleep with almost exclusively slow brain waves. It is also difficult to wake up from this sleep. Both stages of deep sleep are important for feeling refreshed afterward. If these stages are too short, sleep will not feel satisfying.
- Rapid eye movement (REM) sleep: Accounts for about 20% of sleep time in adults and is associated with dreaming. The function of dreaming is not fully understood but appears to be important in the creation of long-term memories. During REM sleep, breathing becomes fast and irregular, heart rate and blood pressure rise, eyes move rapidly, and muscles are immobile. The first cycle has a shorter phase of REM, and as time spent sleeping increases, deep sleep stages decrease and REM sleep increases.

Polysomnography studies have shown that caffeine affects sleep in a dose–response manner—meaning that the effects increase with the size of the dose—but can be detected with doses as low as 1 mg/kg. In particular, caffeine reduces total sleep time and the duration of stages 3 and 4. REM sleep is apparently not altered by caffeine. Depending on when the caffeine was consumed in relation to going to bed, it may or may not affect sleep latency (the time taken to fall to sleep). If taken right before going to bed, caffeine may not alter the ability to fall asleep, but if taken earlier with time for absorption and an increase in blood caffeine concentrations, it is likely to increase the time it takes for sleep to occur.

One study examined the effect of chronic caffeine use to induce insomnia, providing a 400 mg dose of caffeine three times a day (8 a.m., 4 p.m., and 11 p.m.) for a week. Compared with baseline sleep patterns, there was a decrease in total sleep time and stage 4 sleep, and there was an increase in the time taken to fall asleep. REM sleep was not affected. Over the week, a partial tolerance to caffeine developed and changes to sleep patterns lessened. Clearly, athletes need to consider their caffeine use in everyday life and around competition times to ensure that their habits do not degrade their performances.

We all know, of course, that caffeine reduces sleepiness, increases alertness and mental functioning, and enhances performance when people are tired. This can be extremely useful in situations where people are sleep deprived either acutely (one bad night) or chronically (e.g., new baby, fast-lane lifestyle), have extended wakefulness (e.g., doctors on duty), or have to shift their sleep phases (e.g., international travel or shift work). This is usually considered to be achieved by reversing the impairments caused by lack of sleep. The more important questions are whether caffeine adds benefits other than restoring deficits caused by sleep loss and whether it can enhance all these activities without a background of sleep loss or shift in sleep phase.

These questions are hard to answer emphatically because many studies have introduced artifacts or inconsistencies into the research design. The first issue is how well basal sleepiness has been controlled for in study volunteers—an issue that is generally not considered between subjects or within trials in most studies, including those of caffeine and sports performance. In fact, in one of our own studies, undertaken in a group of elite swimmers, we collected information on sleep during the night after a caffeine trial. After we finished, we were stunned to find how late the athletes went to bed, presumably representing their normal patterns; at best they would get 7.5 hours of sleep before their morning workout. Studies of athletes' sleep have shown that many either have poor sleep habits in general or difficulties with sleep in relation to exercise. This might predispose the athletes to higher levels of basal sleepiness and degraded performance, or at least mental and cognitive performance. Such athletes would be likely to respond better to caffeine as a treatment. This needs to be studied in itself as well as controlled for in research design.

There are some final issues to consider with caffeine, sleep, performance, and research. A disadvantage of requiring subjects to withdraw from caffeine in the days leading up to a performance or research trial is that it may add rebound sleepiness to the mix of preperformance effects. As discussed in chapter 9, withdrawal from caffeine is not considered necessary to increase the benefits to performance, so this chance of messing around with sleepiness levels provides another reason not to alter habits leading into an important test or event. And to top it all off, the time of the day may also alter the effects of caffeine, at least on cognitive performance. The circadian rhythms of sleepiness increase around midday, so it is likely that the alerting effects of caffeine taken in the morning and up until midday are greater than when caffeine is taken in the evening.

The athlete's first option should always be to preserve the quality and quantity of sleep. However, there may be competition situations where shortened or interrupted sleep is unavoidable or par for the course for all competitors. In these situations, caffeine may salvage performance from effects of sleep deprivation. This is the best role of caffeine, and several studies related to the military have confirmed that it rescues performance in the short term in soldiers who have had limited sleep. There are also some studies that are more targeted to sports performance where caffeine has enhanced the performance of athletes who are either sleep deprived or not fully recovered from a previous exercise task. In one study, professional rugby players were divided into groups that were either sleep deprived (<6 hours sleep) or not (>8 hours) and received either 4 mg/kg of caffeine or a placebo. They were then required to undertake resistance exercise to volitional fatigue. Sleep deprivation reduced the total load lifted during the workout. Caffeine increased the workout output in both groups, with a greater result seen in the sleep-deprived group.

Of course, such caffeine rescue should not become a long-term solution. It is nevertheless part of the mix that needs to be considered in developing a personal caffeine plan. One further issue needs to be discussed, and that is the vicious cycle that may develop where caffeine use interrupts sleep at night, sleepiness during the day then leads to excessive caffeine use, and so on. An element that can further degrade the situation is the introduction of sleeping tablets into the mix. Sleeping tablets may help ensure sleep in the athlete's everyday life, but they have become an issue in the postcompetition situation. Two particular scenarios come to mind—the athlete who is competing late at night and the athlete who is competing over several days and needs to recover between events. After the hustle and bustle of a day of competition, media interviews, drug tests, and postevent recovery strategies, it can be hard to unwind and fall asleep right away. Being away from the familiarity of home or coping with jet lag can also be part of the story.

In any case, recent publicity regarding the use of sleeping pills by athletes has created discussion and public outcry. It is beyond the scope of this book to discuss the medical and health issues involved with various sleeping medications. However, the topic is important to discuss because, in the public mind if not reality, caffeine is implicated as a factor in the use of these medications. This may occur because the athlete has used caffeine as an ergogenic aid for the competition, or it may occur because the athlete has resorted to caffeine to perk up following the grogginess associated with the sleeping tablet from the previous night. How much caffeine has contributed to the sleep problems that led to the use of the sleeping tablet can't be easily determined. After all, we have pointed out a number of other contributing factors that may interfere with sleep after strenuous competition. Nevertheless, there is evidence that some athletes abuse sleeping tablets and that caffeine use may need to be considered in unraveling the situation.

This scenario of sleeping-tablet abuse also occurs in everyday life for sedentary people, who should also seek medical advice to address or rebalance the situation. It can be more difficult for athletes to get the balance right, however, because they have more factors to add to the equation, as well as the weight of expectations and scrutiny of the media and public. Ultimately, this should be a matter for athletes to resolve with the assistance of their sports medicine teams. However, public reaction and the role-model requirement have necessitated the development of official policies by some sporting agencies, as described in Anatomy of a Caffeine Controversy, Part 2.

# Anatomy of a Caffeine Controversy, Part 2

Two recent examples from Australia have involved a real concern mixed with public outcry over the vicious cycle of sleep and caffeine use in sport. In 2010, a professional Australian rules football player was admitted to a hospital intensive care unit after allegedly suffering side effects due to the consumption of sleeping pills and alcohol after a night football match. Though the media spotlight focused on the specific actions of the player, who was known to be a recovering drug addict, the incident brought to light claims that football players were taking sleeping pills to combat poor sleep associated with caffeine use as well as postgame arousal following night games.

The player, Ben Cousins, acknowledged he had made an error of judgment in taking too many of the sleeping tablets prescribed for him: "I guess it's probably a lesson for everybody. It's not just the medication that you're taking but in particular how much of it. It's been a big wake-up call for me." He stated that he would not continue to take this medication: "No I won't, once bitten, twice shy. It's a serious thing and something I've got to continue to reevaluate. " But he denied that there was a problem with the abuse of caffeine tablets in the Australian Football League (AFL). "A cup of coffee does virtually the same thing. I don't see it as a problem. I haven't seen it abused and I think to abuse caffeine probably has an adverse effect on your performance."

Administrators from the football league acknowledged that the use of caffeine tablets by professional football players was a negative look for the game but stated its context within professional sport:

> **Adrian Anderson, AFL football manager:** "We've spoken to our medical officers who monitor these things through the Australian Sports Anti-Doping Authority doping control forms. They say it's extremely rare that an AFL player would take caffeine . . . and take sleeping tablets." He said that fans and amateur players should remember that AFL players were given medication, including sleeping tablets, under proper medical supervision.

In 2012, the coach of former distance swimmer Grant Hackett declared that Grant's failure to win a third successive gold medal in the 1500 m freestyle event at the Beijing Olympic Games was due to a "lack of clarity" in the race arising from his dependence on the sleeping drug Stilnox (also known as Ambien). In the months leading into the London Olympics, there was much discussion of the use of sleeping tablets, prescribed by official team doctors or personal physicians, by elite athletes. A lot of this discussion occurred in the media and social media and included hype and false information on both sides of the argument. Fortunately, discussion also occurred to good effect within the medical and administrative teams that support high-performance sport. The Australian Olympic Committee

(AOC) produced a policy to promote best practice for the use of sleeping products that could be provided to members of the Australian team at the London Olympics.

Within the discussions, several factors were identified as part of the landscape of the abuse rather than good use of sleeping medications. Caffeine rated plenty of mentions.

> **John Coates, AOC president:** "We have also decided that we will better highlight the practice guidelines . . . in respect to the use of caffeine because we are very worried about the vicious cycle of athletes taking caffeine as a performance enhancer and then needing to take drugs such as Stilnox to get to sleep."

The degree to which caffeine use for competition contributes to the sleep problem, or more importantly, how much an evidence-based use of caffeine in competition would contribute to a sleep problem, is never easy to assess in our multifactorial world. But you can bet that it will always be part of the perception.

Sources: M. Levy and S. Spits, 2010, "'Nothing illegal' in pill drama: Cousins," *The Age*, Melbourne, Australia, July 7, 2010. [Online]. Available: www.theage.com.au/afl/afl-news/nothing-illegal-in-pill-drama-cousins-20100707-zzn3.html [March 4, 2013]; B. English, 2012, "Grant Hackett introduced to Stilnox back in 2003," *News Limited,* July 3, 2012. [Online]. Available: www.news.com.au/sport/london-olympics/drugs-cost-grant-hackett-gold-in-beijing-says-coach-denis-cotterell/story-fndpu6dv-1226415392873 [March 4, 2013]; J. Rakic, 2012, "AOC confirms ban on sleeping tablets," *The Age*, Melbourne, Australia, July 3, 2012. [Online]. Available: www.theage.com.au/olympics/news-london-2012/aoc-confirms-ban-on-sleeping-tablets-20120703-21efw.html [March 4, 2013].

## The Bottom Line

Being an athlete is a 24–7 job. Attention needs to be paid to the times between exercise sessions and the big-picture goals of health, preparation, adaptation, and recovery. Caffeine use, whether for social or ergogenic purposes, should be assessed in terms of big-picture goals as well as any immediate impact on performance. Although the negative impact of caffeine on hydration is now seen as overstated, and the effects on immune status, refueling, and body composition are equivocal, the effect on sleep patterns is an important consideration. Athletes need the benefits of good sleep even more than the rest of the population, but they may squander this precious recovery tool by their injudicious caffeine use.

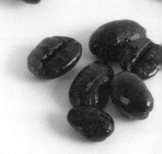

# Individual Considerations
# for Caffeine Use

E xercise physiologists and sport dietitians try to produce guidelines and recommendations for everything that an athlete may need to know about, whether it's training principles, eating plans, recovery strategies, or supplement use. However, the one thing that we know for sure is that human beings are extremely variable in their responses to just about everything. Although general principles are good for a crowd, they may not work for a specific person. At the end of the day (and well before an important competition), it's up to each athlete to try everything out and fine-tune an individualized plan.

## Individual Variability

Because no two humans are exactly alike, everybody responds a little differently to any activity or intervention. In the case of drugs and druglike substances such as caffeine, responses are likely to be even more variable. To provide an example of this, we can look at results of one of our earliest studies of caffeine use, undertaken in the laboratory at the University of Guelph. Back around 1990, we asked well-trained runners to run and cycle as long as they could manage at 80% to 85% $\dot{V}O_2$max, a reasonably high proportion of their aerobic capacity. Each participant did two trials on a lab bike and two on a treadmill, without receiving any information on the time that had elapsed or any other external cues. In each case, one trial followed the consumption of a placebo capsule and the other followed a large dose of caffeine (9 mg/kg) taken 1 hour before exercise. This was back in the early days of caffeine research when we wanted to make sure we saw a result.

We get criticized for undertaking research on caffeine and performance with our athletes. People say we are just encouraging them to use caffeine and that's not good. But any projects that we have done have led to reduced caffeine intake by athletes—fewer athletes using it on fewer occasions in smaller doses. We've been able to help athletes focus on the latest insights and sound uses of the lowest effective doses of caffeine rather than antiquated ideas or the "more is better" approach to caffeine. Even so, it makes many people hot under the collar.

*Sports dietitian to elite athletes*

And see results we did. Figure 9.1 demonstrates that although there was a consistent benefit associated with caffeine intake—all subjects increased their endurance—the variability in the improvement was large, ranging from a 5% to 87% increase in the running trials and from a 10% to 156% increase in the cycling trials!

Clearly, caffeine creates variable outcomes in terms of endurance, but what about performance? A study from Canterbury

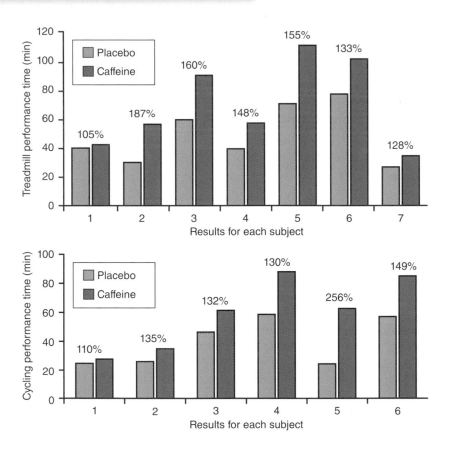

**Figure 9.1**  Effect of 9 mg/kg caffeine on time to exhaustion while running or cycling at ~85% V̇O$_2$max. Results are seen for individual subjects.

Reprinted from T.E. Graham and L.L. Spriet, 1991, "Performance and metabolic responses to a high caffeine dose during prolonged exercise," *Journal of Applied Physiology* 71(6): 2292-2298.

Christ Church University in the United Kingdom investigated caffeine and a simulated 1 km track cycling time trial (the kilo), detailing the results of performance changes in individual subjects. Figure 9.2 summarizes the results of this trial, in which 5 mg/kg caffeine were consumed 75 minutes before the effort compared with a placebo trial. The mean result was an improvement by about 3% (equivalent to 2.3 seconds), but the experience ranged from a small backward step in one person to an improvement of nearly 6% in another.

Some of this variability can be attributed to a myriad of reasons that cause all athletes to have a good day or a bad one any time they put on their training shoes. We try to control for these factors in studies, but you can't get rid of them totally. But there is also growing awareness of, and some explanations for, individuality in the way we metabolize and respond to caffeine. Let's go back to the University of Guelph in 1990. In this study, we asked our athletes to test out the effects of caffeine twice—on bikes and on the treadmill. Figure 9.1 shows that there was some consistency in their variability. For example, subject 1 showed himself to be a smaller responder than the others.

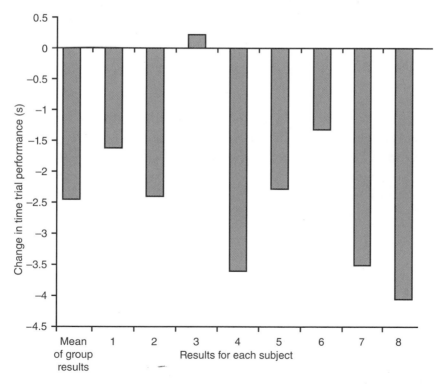

**Figure 9.2** Effect of 5 mg/kg caffeine on performance of a simulated 1 km cycling time trial. Results are seen for mean outcomes and individual subjects.

Adapted, with permission, from W.D. Wiles, D. Coleman, M. Tegerdine, and I.L. Swaine, 2006, "The effects of caffeine ingestion on performance time, speed and power during a laboratory-based 1 km cycling time-trial," *Journal of Sports Sciences* 24(11): 1165-1171.

Every time I take caffeine, I get a caffeine low rather than a caffeine high. It's always been like this—even as a teenager having a can of Coke. It gives me the shakes and inside I feel like I lose equilibrium. I tried Red Bull before a race once, and while I was on the blocks, I felt totally out of it. Even in my civilian life, the closest I get to caffeine is chocolate milk.

*World Championship medalist and Olympian in hurdling*

Now that we are examining the human genome, we can find many examples of small differences in the versions that we have of the same gene. These are known in the business as SNPs (pronounced "snips"), which stands for *single nucleotide polymorphisms*. With regard to caffeine, scientists have identified alterations in the genes for the cytochrome P450 liver enzyme system, which breaks down caffeine, creating fast versus slow caffeine metabolizers. There are also differences in the type and density of distribution of adenosine receptors, which means that some people may have tissues that are more responsive to caffeine than other people have. One gene even seems to code for whether we will tend to develop large or small caffeine habits.

This genetic research is still in its early days but it's beginning to be applied to some of the studies of sports performance. For example, one of the investigations of caffeine and tennis performance reviewed in chapter 5 (table 5.4) divided its group of tennis players into two subsets, depending on the version they carried of a particular gene related to the cytochrome P450 family. It found some evidence of a different physiological response to caffeine in one subset (i.e., they recorded an increase in heart rate following the caffeine dose), although both groups improved their tennis performance equally. In the future, genetic tests may help to predict or explain how we might respond to caffeine use in our sporting activities. But, it will still be of interest to know if there are other controllable factors that can explain variable outcomes from caffeine use.

## Use Habits

There does not seem to be a consistent difference in the performance effects of acute caffeine use between people who are regular caffeine consumers and those who are nonusers. Well-controlled studies from the early 1990s that examined the effects of caffeine on endurance reported no relationship between habitual caffeine consumption and caffeine-induced improvement in exercise capacity. For example, in the study reported in figure 9.1, two athletes were nonusers of caffeine, two were moderate users (120-150 mg/d) and two consumed large amounts of caffeine every day (450-720 mg/d). Yet all of the athletes improved their endurance directly after ingesting a high dose of caffeine.

A follow-up study investigated eight well-trained cyclists, of whom two were nonusers, three were moderate users (<200 mg/d), and three were heavier users (500-940 mg/d). Cycling outcomes improved for all subjects with 3 and 6 mg/kg and for most subjects with the 9 mg/kg dose, independent of habitual caffeine consumption. In a third study, where recreational athletes were asked to cycle to exhaustion at 80% to 85% $\dot{V}O_2$max, one subject was a heavy caffeine user (600 mg/d), two were mild users (180-250 mg/d), and five were nonusers (<50 mg/d). Again, habitual caffeine use had no effect on the ability of caffeine to improve performance (figure 9.3).

Some studies have suggested that the ergogenic effect of caffeine is greater in nonusers versus users of caffeine. For example, one study found that the improvement in exercise time to exhaustion at 80% $\dot{V}O_2$max was greater in a group of 8 nonusers (<50 mg/d) than in another group of 13 users (>300 mg/d). But these findings tend to be the exception rather than the rule.

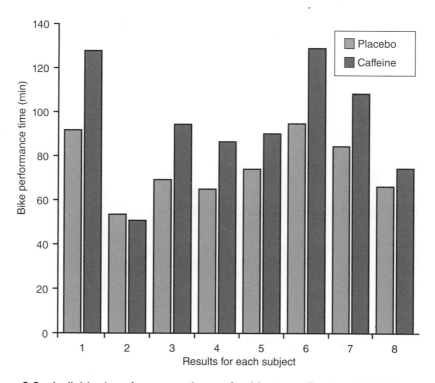

**Figure 9.3**   Individual performance times of subjects cycling to exhaustion at ~80% maximal $O_2$ uptake ($\dot{V}O_2$max) after placebo or caffeine ingestion. Subject 5 was a heavy caffeine user (600 mg/d), subjects 4 and 6 were mild users (180-250 mg/d), and the others were not caffeine users (<50 mg/d).

Reprinted from L.L. Spriet, D.A. MacLean, D.J. Dyck, et al., 1992, "Caffeine ingestion and muscle metabolism during prolonged exercise in humans," *American Journal of Physiology - Endocrinology and Metabolism* 262(6): E891-E898.

# Caffeine Withdrawal

The most common question we get asked about using caffeine for competition is whether the effects are better if athletes have removed caffeine from their daily routines for a number of days, thus receiving an extra shock to the system on competition day when they reintroduce it. It sounds plausible, and in fact, it is standard practice in most studies of caffeine and performance to make subjects withdraw from all dietary sources of caffeine for 1 to 3 days before undertaking each trial. We often hear of athletes who go cold turkey without caffeine for heroic periods—a month, even—before an important race.

The plausibility comes from understanding how caffeine works in our bodies, as described to those who made it through chapter 2. You will remember that we described the ability of caffeine to bind to adenosine receptors, found in so many parts of the body, and block the action that adenosine would have taken. Chronic consumption of caffeine and removal of caffeine from normal use change the availability or activity of those receptors, so the sudden reintroduction of caffeine could be expected to have a different effect. Studies that have monitored the effects of habituating, withdrawing, and reintroducing caffeine on the metabolic responses created by caffeine have shown contradictory findings, but there is a leaning toward the idea that metabolic responses to caffeine could differ with the various scenarios. Of course, athletes don't care about keeping track of metabolism. The bottom line is, will manipulating caffeine intake in the days leading into a race change the effect on performance?

We think the best answer to this question comes from a study conducted by one of us (BD) that used a modern, real-world design—using well-trained athletes, using the moderate caffeine doses now seen as optimal, and measuring performance as the number one goal. The study also took the psychological effect out of the equation by not letting the subjects know for sure if they had given up caffeine or not in the pretrial buildup. Here's how it worked.

Twelve well-trained male cyclists, who were caffeine consumers, were recruited for the study. A double-blind, placebo-controlled crossover design was employed, involving four experimental trials (i.e., all subjects undertook all four trials). The important aspect of this study was that all participants abstained from all dietary caffeine sources for 4 days before the trials—that is, they gave up their lattes and cola drinks. However, during the 4 days, they were given a capsule in the morning and another in the afternoon containing either a placebo or caffeine (to a daily total of 1.5 mg/kg). This was done to standardize the participants' daily habitual intake as either nothing (an unrecognized cold turkey) or 1.5 mg/kg. On day 5, 90 minutes after consuming more capsules containing a placebo or caffeine (3 mg/kg), they did a cycling time trial of 1 hour. Hence, the study was designed to compare withdrawal–placebo, withdrawal–caffeine, no withdrawal–placebo, and no withdrawal–caffeine conditions.

Performance time significantly improved after prerace caffeine ingestion by 1:49 ± 1:41 minutes (3.0%, $p$ = .021) following a withdrawal period and by 2:07 ± 1:28 minutes (3.6%, $p$ = .002) following the nonwithdrawal period. The differences in how well the race-day caffeine worked weren't significant. From this we concluded that the moderate (3 mg/kg) dose of caffeine significantly improved cycling performance and that a 4-day withdrawal period made no difference to its efficacy.

The bottom line seems to be that if you are a regular caffeine user and also use caffeine as a competition aid, you need to determine for yourself whether there is any benefit from withdrawal from caffeine for a day or two before the event. The science would predict that it doesn't matter. But there may be individual differences to the response, and athletes may have a psychological preference. Some of us like to add mystery and effort to important events, so the act of withdrawing from caffeine beforehand is part of the theatrics of competition. On the other hand, many people experience such misery from the loss of their caffeine-consuming rituals or from the physical symptoms of caffeine withdrawal (headaches, grouchiness, sleepiness or loss of alertness) that the idea of missing out on caffeine for a couple of days is abhorrent. See The Perceived Value of Caffeine Withdrawal for further discussion.

## The Perceived Value of Caffeine Withdrawal

Why do most studies of caffeine and performance include a caffeine-withdrawal period in their methodological design, even if we don't think it makes a difference to the performance effects of the caffeine? If we are being honest, it's because scientists often follow each other like sheep—no one wants to have a study criticized during the review process before publication because it doesn't follow scientific convention. Thus, scientists continue to add this burden to their studies because they don't want to rock the boat or have their study perceived as not being rigorously conducted. Similarly, athletes are often superstitious or conscious of the "no pain, no gain" principle. So, they continue to withdraw from caffeine because they are afraid to not follow a habit or custom, or they are afraid that if they don't make sufficient sacrifices, they won't reap the greatest rewards.

It does sometimes seem that caffeine withdrawal makes subjects do better in their study performance or real-life athletes have a blinder of a race. But it could also be that because the withdrawal makes people feel so bad, the reintroduction of caffeine seems to be more magical. In other words, it could just be perception—caffeine allows you to go two steps forward by itself, but if you go one step backward as a result of a caffeine withdrawal, it can allow you to go three steps forward. Either way, you get to the same place. Nevertheless, whether you want to do a scientific trial with grouchy subjects or prepare for a big race, feeling sick and grumpy the day before may be negotiable.

## Length of Effect

Most studies have examined the effects of caffeine on exercise performance about 1 hour after caffeine ingestion. However, some evidence suggests that the performance-enhancing effect lasts considerably longer. Two studies have shown that caffeine ingestion produced ergogenic effects that were evident at 1 hour after intake and persisted for at least 3 hours. This effect was present in groups of caffeine users and nonusers who consumed 5 mg/kg. This result may not be that surprising considering the plasma caffeine levels were similar at 1 and 3 hours postingestion in both groups. At 6 hours, performance was still improved in the nonuser group but not the caffeine users, even though the plasma caffeine level had decreased to the same level in both groups. This information might be of use to athletes who compete in lengthy events or in several events in the same day, so further research is encouraged.

## Timing Intake

The timing of a caffeine dose is of interest to many athletes, including those just mentioned. Several studies have tried to examine this issue, comparing protocols as varied as a single dose before exercise, a single dose during exercise, and repeated doses throughout a single long exercise bout. The general finding is that many protocols work equally well. We found such an outcome in our studies of cola drinks versus caffeine supplements in cycling (see chapter 5). It thus seems that athletes may have several options in designing their optimal protocol of caffeine use. Experience may help to dictate what works best, and the outcome may be based simply on personal preferences or opportunities rather than a superior performance effect. Experimentation and fine-tuning may be needed to develop an individualized approach.

One interesting study required male caffeine users to ride as long as possible at ~80% $\dot{V}O_2$max (~25 minutes) in the morning and again 6 hours later in the afternoon. On one occasion, when they received a placebo in both the morning and afternoon, the performance was identical between the two trials. On a second occasion, they received a placebo in the morning and the caffeine in the afternoon, and performance was improved by the caffeine. On a third occasion, they received a caffeine dose of 5 mg/kg in the morning and 2.5 mg/kg in the afternoon, and the performance effect of caffeine seen in the morning was still present in the afternoon, despite a smaller caffeine dose. On a fourth occasion, when they received a caffeine dose of 5 mg/kg in the morning and a placebo in the afternoon, performance was improved in the morning but surprisingly was still enhanced in the afternoon, despite no additional caffeine.

One way to interpret these data is that you often don't need a dose of caffeine before the session to improve performance at the end of long exercise tasks (2 hours or longer). In fact, if consuming caffeine before longer exercise sessions makes you anxious or overaroused, it might make sense to delay caffeine intake until during the workout. You may even get the same benefit from a lower dose that is delayed. However, if the task is short and there is no opportunity to consume caffeine during the session, the only option is to take the caffeine beforehand. In both of these scenarios, the effect of caffeine ingestion may last for several hours and may benefit a second session of exercise that is undertaken later in the day. This may be useful for the athlete who has several races or bouts in a competition day or several workouts during training. Again, the take-home message is to experiment with the various options and figure out the plan that works best for the individual athlete.

# Method of Intake: Caffeine, Coffee, and Caffeinated Gum

Although most athletes equate caffeine with coffee, scientists rarely use coffee as the method of caffeine administration in research studies. A well-publicized study compared the effects of a caffeine dose of 4.5 mg/kg taken in pure capsule form versus in two mugs of strong coffee. Although the blood caffeine responses were identical, the caffeine in capsule form resulted in the usual metabolic and performance-enhancing effects, but the ingested coffee produced less of a response in plasma epinephrine concentration and little or no effect on endurance (time to exhaustion in an exercise test). It was suggested that the hundreds of additional chemicals in coffee may have negated the usual ergogenic benefit of caffeine alone. Otherwise, the explanation for these results is unclear, and no other studies have reported similar findings to date.

In fact, there are several studies where caffeine consumed in the form of coffee has been associated with significant performance benefits, particularly when the exercise protocol mimicked a sporting event by requiring subjects to complete a time trial rather than ride or run to exhaustion. For example, as summarized in chapter 5 (table 5.2), one study compared the effects of consuming 5 mg/kg of caffeine in the form of a caffeine powder or instant coffee before a cycling protocol that finished with time trial. Both forms improved performance by more than 4% compared with a placebo or decaffeinated coffee. Another study looked at whether a prerace coffee with a meal several hours before an event would cancel out the effect of caffeine consumed specifically for the competition. This study found a clear benefit from caffeine intake that was unaffected by the prior coffee consumption. It seems reasonable to conclude that the administration of caffeine via coffee is an effective way to ensure the performance-enhancing effects of caffeine, as long as an appropriate dose is consumed. Indeed, many athletes like coffee as a pick-me-up before training sessions and competitions. Our main caveat is that the actual caffeine content of a coffee serving can be variable and unpredictable, even when purchased from the same outlet (see chapter 3). Therefore, to achieve a targeted caffeine dose—neither too much nor too little—it is often safer to choose a source that is more stable and labeled.

A newer method of caffeine supplementation is caffeinated chewing gum, and there is some evidence to demonstrate that this gum can be an effective caffeine source. A comparison of caffeine ingestion in capsules versus chewing gum revealed that caffeine absorption rates were higher or faster with the gum, although the bioavailability was the same between the two methods of delivery. It could be argued that a faster absorption with gum may have advantages in some sport situations, especially if the caffeine is taken later in exercise or during the run of play. Because the caffeine is absorbed through the mucosa in the mouth, it bypasses the gastrointestinal system and minimizes the potential for distress.

A couple of studies of sports performance have associated caffeinated gum with a benefit (see chapter 5). In one study, shot-putters saw benefits to throwing in a training session after ingesting 100 mg of caffeine in gum form, while in another, the administration of 240 mg of caffeine in chewing gum improved cycling performance by reducing the decline in performance of repeated high-intensity sprints. Finally, a comparison of the timing of intake of 300 mg caffeine from chewing gum found that performance of a cycling time trial was enhanced when the gum was chewed just before the start of exercise, but not when taken 1 hour and 2 hours beforehand.

## Trained Versus Untrained

The studies examined in this chapter and in chapter 5 make it clear that caffeine has an ergogenic effect when consumed by athletes who are trained to highly trained. Some of this is because such athletes are generally reliable with the performance of familiar tasks. It is easier to detect small improvements in performance following an intervention if day-to-day variability in performance is tight. However, the question is often asked whether caffeine can improve the performance of the weekend warrior or the athlete who is just returning from a break in training and is way down on conditioning. Do you need to be fit to make caffeine count?

This is hard to answer with scientific accuracy. We simply may not be able to undertake a true test of performance with untrained subjects if they can't reliably reproduce the same exercise performance on a day-to-day basis. Philosophically, too, for both the weekend warrior and the out-of-condition serious athlete, attention to more training, proper diet, and rest should be a higher priority in achieving desired performance improvements before supplements figure large.

However, the powerful effects of caffeine on alertness and motivation and its dampening of pain and the general sensation of effort may still be valuable in athletic training. An improvement in the quantity and quality of training may be appreciated by both the weekend warrior and the returning champion. If we can simply feel better when we exercise on a daily basis, this may help us stay active, moving from the untrained to the recreationally trained category or from demoralized and out of shape to motivated and back in town.

## Sex Differences

Studies of caffeine and exercise performance have nearly always been undertaken on male subjects or a mix of men and a few women. This seeming lack of interest in female athletes is because it is often difficult to recruit women of the same caliber of athletic performance or commitment as men. However, in the studies that have reported individual exercise performance data in mixed-sex groups, it appears that the women and men both responded by improving performance following caffeine ingestion.

There has been little systematic study of the specific response of females to caffeine ingestion during exercise. The common excuse for this oversight is the difficulty in studying women. Recruiting women for a study usually results in subjects who are on birth control medication, have regular menstrual cycles, are amenorrheic, or fall in categories in between. Controlling for the presence and phase of the menstrual cycle is a major hassle that sport scientists often simply avoid. Even when a group of female subjects are all eumenorrheic or all on birth control, there is the problem of only being able to test on the days corresponding to the standardized phase of the menstrual cycle.

However, when examining the little information that does exist for women, there do not appear to be major differences in their caffeine-induced responses to exercise and performance when compared with men. For example, a comparison of the effect of sex and exercise on blood concentrations of caffeine revealed similar effects in response to the ingestion of a caffeine dose equal to 6 mg/kg. Two studies from scientists from RMIT University in Australia reported significant improvements in time to complete a 2,000 m rowing task on a Concept 2 rowing ergometer in male and female rowers. The studies, one on female rowers and the other on male rowers, were similar in design and undertaken with rigor. Compared with performance after taking a placebo, caffeine ingestion of 6 mg/ kg and 9 mg/kg improved rowing time by 0.7% and 1.3% in the women, while the mean improvement for the men was 1.2% at both doses. Though there is no expectation that female athletes would respond in a significantly different manner from males to the ingestion of caffeine in sport, further studies need to be done to confirm this hypothesis.

# Use of Other Supplements With Caffeine

Many athletes develop a systematic competition nutrition plan that integrates a number of strategies involving food, sport foods, or supplements. (Of course, many other athletes simply follow a hit-and-miss plan involving a random mixture of things that have no real evidence base, but that's a whole other story.) Optimizing the competition plan requires consideration of whether there is any interaction between the elements—in our case, whether the consumption of caffeine will have any impact on the use of other evidence-based sport supplements or vice versa. Several outcomes could occur; for example, the activity of one supplement could alter, cancel out, or add to the other, or it could even multiply the benefits through synergism. Knowledge of these interactions might lead to reconsideration of the timing or quantity of doses, or even a step back further, of whether it is a good idea to combine the elements at all.

Unfortunately, investigations of the interaction of supplements and sports performance are rare, particularly when it comes to studies including the characteristics we described in chapter 5. This is definitely an overlooked area of sport nutrition research, but we can understand that sport scientists are focused on finding out whether one thing works before they add in other complicating factors. Nevertheless, there are a few areas in which supplement combinations involving caffeine have been examined.

## Carbohydrate and Caffeine

The interaction between carbohydrate intake and caffeine supplementation is important to consider for endurance events, team sports, and racket events because each nutrition strategy, by itself, has a strong potential for performance enhancement in these competition scenarios. An early hypothesis and study promoted the idea that it might not be useful to combine caffeine supplementation with strategies to increase carbohydrate availability for prolonged events. This was underpinned by the original thinking that an important mechanism of caffeine was to increase the mobilization of fatty acids as a fuel source for exercise, sparing muscle glycogen stores. Because carbohydrate intake was known to suppress free fatty acid release, it was felt that including it in pre-event meals or during the event would counteract the beneficial effects of caffeine. Indeed, a study showed that a high carbohydrate diet and prerace meal negated the expected increase in plasma free fatty acids following caffeine ingestion during 2 hours of exercise at ~75% $\dot{V}O_2$ max. Although performance wasn't measured in this study, the authors speculated that the carbohydrate meal had knocked out the value of caffeine supplementation.

We now know that glycogen sparing is not a universal or important part of the way caffeine influences performance of endurance sports, so the carbohydrate counterattack on caffeine is no longer given credibility in this way. In fact, a large number of studies have shown that caffeine enhances performance in athletes who have consumed a high-carbohydrate meal before undertaking an exercise trial. Caffeine supplementation is also able to enhance performance in exercise tasks in which carbohydrate is consumed during the session. However, the magnitude of the benefits of adding caffeine to these sessions seems less than when carbohydrate isn't consumed.

In chapter 5, we discussed a meta-analysis in which the effect of caffeine on the performance of prolonged exercise had been compared between studies and trials in which carbohydrate was consumed and others in which it wasn't. Numerically, caffeine seemed to have a larger influence on performance in the absence of carbohydrate intake during the session. We noted that this doesn't mean that carbohydrate reduces the effect of caffeine, but more likely carbohydrate helps to reduce the development of fatigue over the exercise task. Because the effectiveness of caffeine may be related to how much it can mask the development of fatigue, it could be that carbohydrate-supported sports are more resistant to fatigue and don't need so much rescuing. In other words, the combination is better than either alone, but the benefits of each strategy overlap a little rather than add straight on top of each other.

## Creatine and Caffeine

Creatine supplementation is a popular and evidence-based practice that allows athletes to increase their muscle stores of phosphocreatine, a compound that provides a rapid source of fuel for short, high-intensity bouts of exercise. The benefits of this chronically consumed supplement are generally seen in terms of enhanced ability to undertake workouts involving repeated high-intensity exercise with short recovery intervals (think weight training) as well as improved competition performance of intermittent high-intensity exercise (think team sports). Therefore, there has been some interest in the suggestion that acute use of caffeine may interact with the beneficial effects of creatine loading. The combination of acute caffeine intake in a creatine-loaded athlete might occur in the cases of bodybuilders who take caffeine before a workout to enable themselves to train harder or football players who are looking for multiple ways to reduce the decline in their ability to produce repeat sprint efforts over the course of the match.

The authors of one well-publicized study hypothesized that caffeine ingestion might make creatine supplementation more effective by stimulating creatine transporters in the muscle to increase their uptake of creatine above the effect of creatine supplementation alone. A crossover-designed study tested this out, with each subject completing three trials separated by 3-week washout periods. They consumed a placebo (glucose), creatine, or creatine and caffeine for 6 days during each trial. The creatine dose was ~40 g/d, given in eight equal doses throughout the day, and caffeine was given as a morning dose of 5 mg/kg during the last 3 days of the 6-day creatine-loading procedure. Measurements of the calf muscle tracked changes in creatine concentrations. The ingestion of the placebo had no effects on muscle creatine content or performance of a protocol involving repeated knee extensions before and after the 6 days. The creatine supplementation increased muscle phosphocreatine content slightly and increased exercise capacity. Surprisingly, consuming caffeine in the final 3 days of a creatine protocol completely abolished the improvement in the knee extension protocol seen with creatine alone, even though the increases in muscle phosphocreatine content were still present! In effect, the study produced the concerning result that caffeine intake might counteract the beneficial effects of creatine loading.

There are concerns, however, with the design of this study that might require rethinking the results. This mainly relates to the fact that subjects undertook each of the trials with only a 3-week gap between. Many other studies have shown that once a muscle has become creatine loaded, it takes 6 to 8 weeks for it to wash out—in other words, for the muscle phosphocreatine content to return back to normal levels. Therefore, there may have been some carryover from one treatment to the next. In addition, there was no caffeine-only trial in which we could judge the effect of caffeine on the performance of the knee extension protocol. Furthermore, the reversal of ergogenic effects of creatine loading is difficult to understand in light of the fact that the last caffeine dose was given ~20 hours before the exercise test. It is not clear how the presence of caffeine in the body for 3 days would negate the effects of creatine loading when the increased muscle phosphocreatine content persisted. The authors were unable to present any explanations.

Since this study was published, several other investigations have tried to replicate the findings. None has been able to do so. In fact, one study reported that running exercise time was improved by the acute consumption of caffeine (6 mg/kg) in subjects who had creatine loaded for 6 days. The conclusion is that there is no good evidence to suggest a negative interaction between the ergogenic effects of creatine and caffeine in humans engaged in regular exercise activities.

## Sodium Bicarbonate and Caffeine

The ingestion of sodium bicarbonate in the hours before exercise leads to an increase in blood pH, enhancing the capacity to buffer the increase in hydrogen ions and acidosis that occurs in high-intensity exercise where the anaerobic energy pathways are heavily involved. Numerous reports demonstrate that such bicarbonate loading improves performance during exercise and sporting activities lasting from 2 to 10 minutes. These include rowing, cycling, and swimming races, events that may also benefit from caffeine supplementation. It makes sense to see if the combination of supplements could improve performance more than either of them alone.

Unfortunately, we are currently limited to the results of three studies to test out this interest (see chapter 5 for more details). Although these investigations did not support any benefits of combining the supplements, the results might be seen as specific to the study protocols rather than a universal finding. The first study, for example, involved the performance of two 200 m swimming races held 30 minutes apart, and it found no differences in combined swim times between any of the treatments (placebo, caffeine, sodium bicarbonate, and the combination of the supplements). However, closer examination of the results reveals that differences may have occurred between treatments and between the two races that might have been teased out with a large group of subjects or that might not have been present if a different swimming test had been chosen (after all, at the elite level of swimming it's not often that a competitor would swim two races so close together).

Our interpretation of the results of this study is that caffeine may have helped swimmers to race faster in the first swim, but they paid a penalty for this by swimming more slowly in the second race. However, the addition of bicarbonate may have helped to overcome this inability to back up with a second good performance. At the very least, this study suggests that further work is needed and should include careful thinking about the timing of supplement intake and pacing strategies for high-intensity exercise.

The second study examined 2,000 m rowing performance on a lab ergometer in eight well-trained rowers (six men and two women). Caffeine ingestion alone (6 mg/kg) improved performance by 2%, but the ingestion of sodium bicarbonate alone or in combination with caffeine did not significantly improve performance. In this study, the confounding effect was the gastrointestinal symptoms caused by the bicarbonate loading, a common side effect that may be preventable. Again, manipulating the supplement protocols may produce a strategy in which gut symptoms are minimized, and the two strategies could work together by independent and additive mechanisms—caffeine by affecting the brain and sodium bicarbonate by buffering acid–base changes. Finally, a study of 3 km cycling found that both caffeine and bicarbonate enhanced performance when taken by themselves, but the combination of both did not further improve the outcome. It is possible that bicarbonate loading reduced the fatigue associated with the high-intensity exercise, while caffeine simply masked the effect of this fatigue; therefore, both reached the same outcome by different means.

## The Bottom Line

Many intricate details of individual responsiveness and sport specificity need to be taken into account before caffeine supplementation can be applied to training and competition practices. Sport scientists need to continue to plug away at doing better research to test both fundamental and intricate questions of caffeine and sports performance. In the end, however, the bottom line will come down to the athlete's ability to evaluate whether a caffeine supplementation strategy is right for him or her. So, it is time to conclude this book with some tools to help athletes make these decisions.

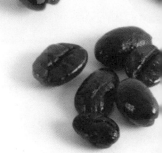

# Chapter

. . . . . . . . . . . . . .

# 10

# Putting It All Together

In the previous chapters, we have tried to gather together an objective account of caffeine use for athletes. This has included the following:

- The history of caffeine in science and sports performance
- An overview of the way caffeine affects the body
- Sources of caffeine in the everyday diet and for specific use in sport
- The latest evidence of the range of sporting events in which caffeine might provide benefits to performance, including the limitations of this research
- The potential harmful effects and side effects of caffeine use
- The ethics of caffeine use in relation to antidoping rules

It is both interesting and troubling that a substance consumed daily by the overwhelming majority of adults to enhance their well-being and daily activities can polarize the community when applied to sport. It is not the intention of this book to promote caffeine use by athletes. Rather, our goal is to provide independent information on caffeine use that can

- help athletes, coaches, or those involved in sporting organizations who are interested in caffeine to make well-informed decisions about whether to use it or support its use, and
- help athletes who already take caffeine in an attempt to enhance sports performance to assess whether they follow best practice (maximum benefits and minimum side effects) in their specific uses.

In finishing, we will attempt to integrate all of this information in a way that achieves our goals. Two themes are needed: promoting an infrastructure in which caffeine can be used appropriately in sport and providing tools to allow people to make their own decisions about caffeine use.

# Help for Organizations:
# Establishing a Framework for Evidence-Based Uses

In chapter 5, we found clear evidence that caffeine intake can enhance the performance of a variety of sports and sporting activities. A new understanding is emerging that a variety of protocols of caffeine intake may be useful and that a threshold of effectiveness may be reached at intakes of ~3 mg/kg. Such intakes, typically ranging from 150 mg for a 50 kg female athlete up to 300 mg for a 100 kg male athlete, fall within the daily caffeine dose described as low-moderate by health authorities and expert panels. Furthermore, they represent doses that can be achieved from a variety of caffeine sources in the general food supply or from specialized sport foods and supplements. They are unlikely to exceed the mean daily intake of caffeine consumed by most adults around the world or to produce meaningful elevations in urinary caffeine concentrations in the samples produced at doping control after events.

Everyone needs to take a deep breath when it comes to one of the footy issues of the week—Australian Football League players taking caffeine tablets and No-Doz before games. . . . I can understand why the AFL doesn't like the image of its players popping caffeine tablets before a game, and perhaps even at halftime in a bid to play at their peak. It clearly doesn't want kids following suit at junior levels, and I reckon that's fair enough. But AFL is a professional sport and clubs and players will always try to seek an edge wherever they can.

*Shane Crawford, former captain of Australian Football League team (2010)*

How caffeine intake enhances sports performance is still not fully understood, but it is typically seen as a reduction in the fatigue or performance decline that would otherwise occur during an event. This principle is similar to the way that people use caffeine in other occupational activities in which fatigue reduces effectiveness (e.g., drivers, pilots, military personnel, students). Most adults develop their own pattern of caffeine intake to enhance their well-being and ability to complete vocational or recreational activities and tasks.

To enhance the effectiveness of caffeine use in sport (i.e., to maximize benefits and minimize side effects), we need further sport-specific research to provide knowledge about optimal protocols for caffeine supplementation. Areas that deserve attention include the following:

- Effects of caffeine supplementation on sports performance under field conditions, including the following key outcomes from such research:
  - Better understanding of effects that are meaningful to the outcome of sport rather than traditional approaches of statistical significance

- Specific protocols that allow caffeine supplementation to be integrated into the practical characteristics of an event (e.g., time-tabling of the event, coordination with pre- and during-event nutrition and hydration)
- Integration of the effects of caffeine supplementation with competition arousal and the external distractions of the competition environment
- Effects of caffeine supplementation in various environments (altitude, temperature, and so on)
- Effects of caffeine on performance of repeated events, including tolerance to repeated episodes of caffeine supplementation
- How chronic use of caffeine to promote training performance affects competition preparation
- Variability of the effects of caffeine supplementation among and within people
- The range of protocols of caffeine intake and sources of caffeine that are safe and effective
- Effects on special populations, including elite athletes, female athletes, adolescent athletes, masters athletes, and athletes with disabilities
- Interactions with other ergogenic nutrients (e.g., carbohydrate, fluid) and supplements (e.g., creatine, bicarbonate, nitric oxide stimulators)
- Effect of caffeine supplementation on performance undertaken with suboptimal preparation (e.g., inadequate sleep, inadequate recovery, restricted energy intake)
- Conditions under which caffeine is harmful to health or performance
- Effect of caffeine on postexercise recovery, including sleep

Better knowledge in these areas could lead to a reduced caffeine intake by athletes. This would include less misuse of caffeine in sport and better targeting of caffeine use to times and protocols in which it is likely to be effective.

In theory, athletes should be able to manage a safe and socially acceptable caffeine intake to prioritize its effect on sports performance within the ethics and rules of their sport. In practice, however, caffeine use in sport continues to be problematic.

This review will conclude with a brief overview of some of the issues illustrated by these episodes, demonstrating the challenges involved in setting up a framework to allow better use of caffeine by athletes.

1. There is evidence that some athletes do use caffeine as an ergogenic aid following best practice (i.e., safe, effective, ethical) and that some science and sports medicine support networks are involved in sound activities related to the research on, education on, and implementation of these supplementation practices.

2. Equally there is evidence that some athletes do not follow best practice or evidence-based protocols for caffeine use in training, competition performance, or social intake of caffeine. At best, these practices are ineffective, but in the worst-case scenario, they may be detrimental to health and performance. Problematic practices include the use of unnecessarily large doses of caffeine in competition and, on some occasions, the use of sleeping aids to combat the subsequent inability to sleep.

3. It is evident that many athletes and coaches are unaware of new information regarding caffeine and sports performance. The culture of sports, including the more-is-better attitude to any intervention, might contribute to poor caffeine supplementation practices and caffeine misuse.

4. Some science and sports medicine practitioners who work with elite athletes or provide commentary to media on these matters are also unaware of current knowledge on caffeine and sports performance. They may contribute both to the reality and the perception of poor caffeine use in sport.

5. It appears that most people learn to organize their caffeine intake to promote well-being and to assist their ability to complete occupational and recreational activities; after all, 90% of adults are regular consumers of caffeine. However, many consumers do not regard caffeine use by athletes as part of this spectrum.

6. Antidoping agencies have provided an environment that is supportive of caffeine research, education, and use by athletes when it is undertaken transparently and involving best practice. The stated position of WADA with relation to caffeine is clear. At times, however, some messages from antidoping agencies related to caffeine use have been confusing (or perhaps have had their intentions altered by media communications).

7. Community members are rightly concerned about caffeine misuse in sport. However, they often also hold emotive views about caffeine that are neither factual nor rational. These views exacerbate the perception of the extent and nature of true problems.

8. A range of projects and approaches is needed to create major change in the current problems of poor caffeine use in sport. Stakeholders include athletes and coaches, science and sports medicine practitioners and their professional bodies, governing bodies of sports, sporting institutes and academies, researchers, regulatory bodies of foods and therapeutic goods, media, antidoping agencies, and the sport-loving community. Additional specialists who may provide expert help to identify and tackle problems include experts in caffeine pharmacology as well as social researchers who could investigate current beliefs and patterns of caffeine use among athletes

and community members. Major solutions may require the involvement of all stakeholders. However, smaller projects and strategies involving targeted sections of sport may be able to test out models that can be later applied to the larger athlete community. We hope that the information presented in this book may be used to develop this infrastructure.

# Help for Athletes and Coaches: Using Caffeine Safely and Effectively

It should be clear by now that response to caffeine is highly individualized. Can it enhance *your* athletic performance? With the knowledge you've gleaned from this text, as well as some tools included in this chapter, you will be guided in safely experimenting with caffeine as an ergogenic aid and assessing its effectiveness for you.

Table 10.1 lists advantages and disadvantages of various methods of caffeine supplementation. With this, you have a handy reference for considering which ways of ingesting caffeine might work well for you—or not work at all.

It will be important to calculate your average intake of caffeine, so you are encouraged to visit www.griffith.edu.au/health/centre-health-practice-innovation/research/nutrition to use our free online caffeine intake calculator. All you need to do is proceed down the list of caffeine-containing foods, noting how frequently you consume them. We usually suggest you consider the past 3 months as your habitual behavior.

South African distance runner Elana Meyer tested positive for excessive levels of caffeine in a 10 km race in Bali in February 2002. Elana won the silver medal in the women's 10,000-meter event at the 1992 Barcelona Olympic Games.

For example, Joe, who lives in the United Kingdom, drinks 1 cup of coffee every day from the coffee shop near work. On the weekend he replaces this with tea. In addition, he eats three chocolate bars per week. Joe would enter all of this information into the tool. This typical pattern of food and fluids means that Joe's average daily caffeine intake is 102 mg with a range of 36 mg to 182 mg. The range is because Joe drinks commercial coffee, which has a variable caffeine concentration.

Table 10.2 is a detailed checklist that will help you assess your current caffeine use, its effects on your health and goals of daily living, and whether there is opportunity or benefit to altering these patterns to assist with training goals. Table 10.3 is a checklist that addresses the specific use of caffeine to promote competition outcomes. These checklists provide a systematic way to undertake

**Table 10.1**   Pros and Cons of Caffeine Sources as Supplements for Sports Performance

| Source | Pros | Cons |
|---|---|---|
| Coffee | • Loved and part of social rituals<br>• Available from many locations<br>• Possibly able to give a dose within the effective range in a practically consumed serving<br>• Provides a source of antioxidants | • Unknown and variable caffeine dose—can be hit and miss<br>• May contain other ingredients that counteract performance-enhancing effects of caffeine |
| Tea | • Enjoyed and part of social rituals<br>• Available from many locations<br>• Provides a good source of antioxidants | • Unknown and variable caffeine dose—can be hit and miss<br>• May not provide a performance-enhancing dose when consumed in usual amounts |
| Iced coffee and frappé-style drinks | • Enjoyed and part of social rituals<br>• Available from many locations<br>• Provide a source of dairy in the overall diet (protein, calcium) and for sport goals (carbohydrate, protein), particularly following exercise | • May be a source of unnecessary fat and sugar in the total diet<br>• Unknown and variable caffeine dose—can be hit and miss<br>• May contain other ingredients that counteract performance-enhancing effects of caffeine |
| Energy drinks | • Popular in certain populations<br>• Generally available<br>• Provide a known dose of caffeine<br>• Provide a dose within the effective range in a practically consumed serving<br>• Could be consumed both before and during exercise (if defizzed)<br>• Provide fluid, carbohydrate, and perhaps other ingredients that are useful for sports performance | • May have a negative image<br>• High in sugar, which may need to be considered in overall dietary goals |
| Cola drinks and other caffeinated soft drinks | • Popular<br>• Widely available<br>• Known dose of caffeine<br>• Can provide a dose within the effective range, especially when consumed throughout prolonged events to meet carbohydrate intake goals, in conjunction with other caffeine sources, or toward the end of a long event when more sensitive to small caffeine doses<br>• Provide fluid and carbohydrate in amounts that are useful for sports performance | • Need to be defizzed before consuming during exercise, which can be time consuming<br>• High in sugar, which may need to be considered in overall dietary goals |
| Caffeinated sport drinks | • Provide a known dose of caffeine<br>• Provide a dose within the effective range, especially when consumed before or throughout prolonged events to meet carbohydrate intake goals or toward the end of a long event when more sensitive to small caffeine doses<br>• Could be consumed both before and during exercise<br>• Provide fluid, carbohydrate, and electrolytes to meet other nutritional needs for sports performance<br>• Manufactured for sports performance and therefore have acceptable reputation for use in sport | • Can be difficult to find in usual commercial outlets<br>• High in sugar, which may need to be considered in overall dietary goals |

| Source | Pros | Cons |
|--------|------|------|
| Caffeinated sport gels and confectionary | • Provide a known dose of caffeine<br>• Can provide a dose within the effective range, especially when consumed before or throughout prolonged events to meet carbohydrate intake goals, in conjunction with other caffeine sources, or toward the end of a long event when more sensitive to small caffeine doses<br>• Manufactured for sports performance and therefore have acceptable reputation for use in sport | • Require significant intake (e.g., at least 2-4 servings) to reach effective dose, which requires intake of a significant amount of carbohydrate |
| Caffeinated gum | • Provides a known dose of caffeine<br>• Can provide a dose within the effective range<br>• Rapidly absorbs through mouth rather than stomach<br>• Some commercial forms come with approval of military health authorities, which may confer a better reputation to its use<br>• Can be used when intake of fluid or carbohydrate is unnecessary or unwanted | • May be easy to overdo the total caffeine dose |
| Preworkout supplements | | • Caffeine dose is often unknown and not stated on label<br>• May contain other stimulants, often also in unknown quantities<br>• May contain stimulants or other substances that are banned in sport |
| Weight-loss supplements containing caffeine | | • Caffeine dose is often unknown and not stated on label<br>• May contain other stimulants, often also in unknown quantities<br>• May contain stimulants or other substances that are banned in sport |
| NoDoz and other over-the-counter medications | • Provide a known dose of caffeine<br>• Can provide a dose within the effective range<br>• Can be used when intake of fluid or carbohydrate is unnecessary or unwanted | • May be easy to overdo the total caffeine dose<br>• Have a poor public perception |

a cost–benefit analysis of present or contemplated caffeine use from a consistent viewpoint: Is it safe? Is it legal? Is it effective? Can I afford it?

Figure 10.1 may be used to analyze the effects of caffeine on your performance as you experiment with different doses, forms, and timing of intake. Depending on your sport, you might like to do this in some key training sessions where you mimic your race plan, you might keep this as a competition record only, or you could combine the two scenarios. The important point is that you should complete this questionnaire as soon after you have finished the session as possible, while the details are fresh in your mind. Of course, you will need to add comments about your post-event sleep patterns the next day. The value of these records is that they will provide you with an objective account of what you tried and how the experience worked (or didn't). Sometimes, it's only when you can systematically piece together the clues from several of these records that the best protocol for your needs will become clear.

We hope that these resources will help you to make good decisions regarding caffeine use so that these decisions can add to the quality of your life and the outcome of your sporting endeavors.

**Table 10.2** Checklist for Assessing Caffeine in the Training Diet

| | Issues | Comments | Tools |
|---|---|---|---|
| What is my present caffeine habit? | What is my daily total caffeine intake? | Assess the caffeine content of your everyday or habitual eating and drinking practices—you may be surprised! | We have created a handy online resource to calculate your average daily caffeine intake (www.griffith.edu.au/health/centre-health-practice-innovation/research/nutrition). It will also give you a minimum and maximum value due to the variability of caffeine from some sources (see Do I Have a Caffeine Addiction? sidebar in chapter 4) |
| | What are my major sources of caffeine? | • Assess the nutritional and practical aspects of the foods, drinks, and supplements that contribute caffeine to your diet.<br>• Consider issues such as the energy content of your caffeine sources and the coincidental intake of healthy (e.g., antioxidants) and harmful ingredients (e.g., excess fat, sugar).<br>• Consider costs and quality control of caffeine sources—is the caffeine content reliable? Are you aware of all other ingredients? | See table 10.1 of the pros and cons of various caffeine sources. |
| | What is the timing of my usual caffeine intake? | • Assess whether your habitual caffeine intake is consumed in a way that may influence training performance (i.e., do you consume caffeine in the hours before a workout or during the session?).<br>• Assess whether your habitual or training-related caffeine intake has an effect on your sleep patterns (i.e., do you consume caffeine in the hours before your bedtime?). | |

(continued)

**Table 10.2** *(continued)*

| | Issues | Comments | Tools |
|---|---|---|---|
| My intended caffeine use for training: Is it safe? | How does my usual caffeine intake fit into the generally recognized bands of caffeine intake? | • Assess where you fit into the caffeine intake spectrum: <br>  • Low: 80-250 mg/d (1.1-3.5 mg/kg) <br>  • Moderate: 300-400 mg/d (4-6 mg/kg) <br>  • High: >400 mg/d (>6-8 mg/kg) <br>• Am I surprised at the total? Should I be cutting down rather than increasing or moving it around in the day? | |
| | Are there any preexisting health concerns that I should be worried about? | • Check with your doctor regarding heart issues or other medical problems that require the avoidance of caffeine. <br>• Note that low intakes of caffeine are likely to be effective for sports performance, and even if you have a clear health record, it is unnecessary to deliberately take large caffeine doses. | |
| | Am I doubling up on intake of stimulants or consuming caffeine in concert with large amounts of alcohol? | • If you are deliberately combining caffeine with other stimulants or alcohol, make sure you are aware of the potential risks. <br>• Note your potential for inadvertent combinations, such as caffeine intake while using over-the-counter cold medications containing pseudoephedrine. | |
| | Is there any evidence that the amount of caffeine that I am consuming is causing any side effects? | • Check your sleep patterns. Are the quality and quantity of your sleep affected by the total caffeine intake over the day or timing of intake later in the day? <br>• Check to see if you are showing any signs of caffeine addiction. There may be benefits to reorganizing your caffeine intake to get on top of this. | See Do I Have a Caffeine Addiction? sidebar in chapter 4. |
| My intended caffeine use for training: Is it legal? | Am I part of a sporting code or sporting environment that prohibits the deliberate use of caffeine to aid sports performance? | • The WADA antidoping code does not prohibit the use of caffeine by athletes in any circumstance. <br>• The NCAA code prohibits caffeine use only when it leads to urinary caffeine levels in excess of 15 µg/ml, which is only likely to be reached with very high intakes that are unnecessary. <br>• Some sport clubs or associations may have their own rules or codes that discourage specific use of caffeine for sports performance. Even though this may be hard to police, athletes and coaches need to understand the context of these rules. | |

| | Issues | Comments | Tools |
|---|---|---|---|
| My intended caffeine use for training: Is it effective? | • Are there workouts that might specifically benefit from caffeine intake?<br>• Is the caffeine dose within the effective range and timing of intake?<br>• Are there opportunities to time the intake of my habitual caffeine use so that it provides an advantage for a workout?<br>• Are there opportunities to practice my competition caffeine strategies? | Sessions that might be targeted:<br>• Key workouts during heavy volume training or high lifestyle fatigue where you need to be able to protect your ability to train at high intensity or with good technique and concentration<br>• Key training sessions where you are also deliberately training low in relation to fuel stores<br>• Workouts simulating your event where you are trialing or fine-tuning competition strategies<br>Effective doses:<br>• ~3 mg/kg total taken before and during lengthy sessions<br>• 1-2 mg/kg taken toward the end of a lengthy session or when fatigued<br>• Simulation of caffeine use for competition | See Can Caffeine Rescue Train-Low Tactics? sidebar in chapter 5.<br><br>See tables 3.1 and 3.2 for doses of caffeine in common caffeine sources.<br><br>See chapter 5 for a summary of studies in which caffeine has been found to be effective.<br><br>See checklist for competition in table 10.3. |
| My intended caffeine use for training: Can I afford it? | • How expensive are the caffeine sources in my diet?<br>• Am I consuming other ingredients that I may not need just to get the caffeine? | • Consider the financial outlay for specialized caffeine sources for use before or in training and whether these are always necessary (outside practicing actual competition strategies). Perhaps there are alternatives.<br>• Consider the intake of other ingredients in the caffeine serving (e.g., sugar, fat). Perhaps there are more suitable sources of caffeine. | |

**Table 10.3**  Checklist for Determining Caffeine for Optimal Competition Performance

| | Issue | Comments | Tools |
|---|---|---|---|
| What caffeine strategies have I tried before in my events? | What is my past experience with caffeine in competition? | • Examine your past attempts to use caffeine in competition settings. Hindsight may not always be possible if the episodes are too far in the past, but use any you can remember.<br>• Start a debrief diary to collect objective information on your new experiences with caffeine and performance in training and events! | Use debrief form for competition caffeine use (figure 10.1). |
| My intended caffeine use for competition: Is it safe? | Are there any preexisting health concerns that I should be worried about? | • Check with your doctor regarding heart issues or other medical problems that require the avoidance of caffeine.<br>• Low intakes of caffeine are likely to be effective for sports performance, and even if you have a clear health record, it is unnecessary to deliberately take large caffeine doses. | |
| | Will my total intake of caffeine for the day of competition stay in the low-moderate range? | • Add up your intended caffeine use in all its forms for the competition bout.<br>• Don't forget to consider any caffeine intake associated with social activities or for additional competition bouts on the same day. | |
| My intended caffeine use for competition: Is it legal? | Am I part of a sporting code or sporting environment that prohibits the deliberate use of caffeine to aid sports performance? | • The WADA antidoping code does not prohibit the use of caffeine by athletes in any circumstances.<br>• The NCAA code prohibits caffeine use only when it leads to urinary caffeine levels in excess of 15 µg/ml, which is only likely to be reached with very high intakes that are unnecessary.<br>• Some sport clubs or associations may have their own rules or codes that discourage specific use of caffeine for sports performance. Even though this may be hard to police, athletes and coaches need to understand the context of these rules. | |

| | Issue | Comments | Tools |
|---|---|---|---|
| My intended caffeine use for competition: Is it effective? | • Am I competing in an event in which there is good evidence that performance might specifically benefit from caffeine intake?<br>• Is the caffeine dose within the effective range and timing of intake?<br>• Have I had opportunities to practice my competition caffeine strategies during previous events or training sessions to fine-tune them? | Sessions that might be targeted:<br>• Endurance sports (>60 min)<br>• Brief sustained high-intensity sports (1-60 min)<br>• Team and intermittent sports—work rates<br>• Team and intermittent sports—skills and concentration<br>Effective doses<br>• 3 mg/kg total taken before and during lengthy sessions<br>• 1-2 mg/kg taken toward the end of a lengthy session or when fatigued | See chapter 5 for a summary of studies in which caffeine has been found to be effective.<br>See tables 3.1 and 3.2 for doses of caffeine in common caffeine sources.<br>Use debrief form for competition caffeine use (figure 10.1). |
| | • Am I competing in an event in which the evidence is unclear that performance might specifically benefit from caffeine intake?<br>• Is the caffeine dose within the effective range and timing of intake for other sports?<br>• Have I had opportunities to practice my competition caffeine strategies during previous events or training sessions to fine-tune them? | Sports in which there is unclear evidence of performance enhancement and require further research:<br>• Skill sports involving low-intensity exercise<br>• Single efforts involving strength or power<br>• Potentially effective doses:<br>• ~3 mg/kg total taken before and during lengthy sessions or before single-effort events<br>• 1-2 mg/kg taken toward the end of a lengthy session or when fatigued | See chapter 5 for a summary of studies and the lack of clear evidence for effective use of caffeine in these sports.<br>See tables 3.1 and 3.2 for doses of caffeine in common caffeine sources.<br>Use debrief form for competition caffeine use (figure 10.1). |
| | Are the sources of caffeine that I intend to use suitable to meet my goals? | Consider the types or combination of caffeine sources that could contribute to your competition protocol. | See table 10.1 for the pros and cons of various caffeine sources. |
| | Are there any individual issues that I need to consider? | Consider the following issues:<br>• Do you feel you benefit or lose by undertaking caffeine withdrawal before undertaking your competition caffeine strategy?<br>• Are you taking other supplements or competition nutrition strategies that need to be integrated with the caffeine protocol?<br>• Do you need to compete more than once in this event? Will you need to consider the timing of the dose to suit several events or the need for recovery between events? | |
| My intended caffeine use for competition: Can I afford it? | Is there any evidence that the amount of caffeine that I am consuming is causing any side effects? | When there is the need to compete on successive days, is the caffeine protocol impairing sleep patterns and recovery between events? | Use debrief form for competition caffeine use (figure 10.1). |

# FIGURE 10.1 DEBRIEF ON CAFFEINE USE IN COMPETITION

Name: _____ Event: _____

Date: _____ Duration: _____

Body weight: _____ Caffeine abstinence: Y / N If yes, when? _____

Competition conditions: _____

| Record of caffeine intake | Before event (timing) | During event (timing) | Caffeine intake (mg) |
|---|---|---|---|
| *Coca-Cola/Pepsi* | | 2 × ~150 ml (5 and 10 km into run) | |
| *PowerBar caffeinated gel* | 1 sachet (40 g) taken 60 min prior | | 25 |
| | | | |
| | | | |
| | | | |
| | | | |
| | | | |
| **Total caffeine intake** | | | mg |
| | | | mg/kg |

## Performance

How well did you perform today as a percentage of your best competition form? _____%

How hard did your effort feel as a percentage of your maximum? _____%

What do you think limited your performance today (e.g., leg tiredness, acute pain, tactical issues, general fatigue, dehydration, lack of fuel, confidence)?

_____

_____

What activities were critical in your competition performance? Rate how you think caffeine affected these activities (only select those relevant to this event).

| | Tick if important | Strongly negative | Negative/ adverse | No effect | Positive/ good | Strongly positive | Unsure |
|---|---|---|---|---|---|---|---|
| Endurance in prolonged exercise (30+ minutes) | | 1 | 2 | 3 | 4 | 5 | 6 |
| Speed and power in prolonged exercise (30+ minutes) | | 1 | 2 | 3 | 4 | 5 | 6 |
| Endurance in short-term, intense exercise | | 1 | 2 | 3 | 4 | 5 | 6 |
| Speed and power in short-term, intense exercise | | 1 | 2 | 3 | 4 | 5 | 6 |
| Strength | | 1 | 2 | 3 | 4 | 5 | 6 |
| Concentration and alertness | | 1 | 2 | 3 | 4 | 5 | 6 |
| Skills | | 1 | 2 | 3 | 4 | 5 | 6 |
| Calming nerves | | 1 | 2 | 3 | 4 | 5 | 6 |

## Side Effects of Caffeine Use

Please note the severity of any side effects as a result of using caffeine for this competition.

| | Barely noticeable | Noticeable but minor | Noticeable | Severe | Very severe | Unsure |
|---|---|---|---|---|---|---|
| Tremors or shakes | 1 | 2 | 3 | 4 | 5 | 6 |
| Headaches | 1 | 2 | 3 | 4 | 5 | 6 |
| Elevated heart rate | 1 | 2 | 3 | 4 | 5 | 6 |
| Increased sweating | 1 | 2 | 3 | 4 | 5 | 6 |
| Increased urine volume | 1 | 2 | 3 | 4 | 5 | 6 |
| Gut discomfort | 1 | 2 | 3 | 4 | 5 | 6 |
| Caffeine addiction | 1 | 2 | 3 | 4 | 5 | 6 |

Please note the frequency (proportion of time) that you experienced any side effects as a result of using caffeine for this competition.

| | Never (0%) | Rarely (<25%) | Occasion-ally (25%-50%) | Regularly (50%-75%) | Almost always (>75%) | Always (100%) | Unsure |
|---|---|---|---|---|---|---|---|
| Tremors or shakes | 1 | 2 | 3 | 4 | 5 | 6 | 7 |
| Headaches | 1 | 2 | 3 | 4 | 5 | 6 | 7 |
| Elevated heart rate | 1 | 2 | 3 | 4 | 5 | 6 | 7 |
| Increased sweating | 1 | 2 | 3 | 4 | 5 | 6 | 7 |
| Increased urine volume | 1 | 2 | 3 | 4 | 5 | 6 | 7 |
| Gut discomfort | 1 | 2 | 3 | 4 | 5 | 6 | 7 |
| Caffeine addiction | 1 | 2 | 3 | 4 | 5 | 6 | 7 |

Other side effects or unusual effects: _____

_____

_____

## Sleep

Did you consume caffeine following this event? Y / N

Amount _____

Did you consume alcohol following this event? Y / N

Amount _____

How long did it take to fall asleep at night after your event? _____

What strategies (if any) did you use to achieve sleep (e.g., sleeping tablets, hot milk)? _____

For how many hours did you sleep? _____

Rate the effect you think caffeine had on the following aspects of your postevent sleep.

| | Strongly negative | Negative/ adverse | No effect | Positive/ good | Strongly positive | Unsure |
|---|---|---|---|---|---|---|
| Length of time to fall asleep | 1 | 2 | 3 | 4 | 5 | 6 |
| Quality of sleep | 1 | 2 | 3 | 4 | 5 | 6 |
| Comparison with normal sleep patterns | 1 | 2 | 3 | 4 | 5 | 6 |

From L. Burke, B. Desbrow, and L. Spriet, 2013, *Caffeine for sports performance* (Champaign, IL: Human Kinetics).

# Appendix

## A Compelling Case of the Issues Involved With Caffeine Doping in Sport

The following is a transcript of an interview between journalist Warwick Hadfield and former Australian modern pentathlete Alex Watson.

**Warwick Hadfield:** In August 1988, a happy and optimistic Alex Watson set off for the Seoul Olympics to compete in the modern pentathlon. This is the sport devised by the father of the modern Olympics, Baron Pierre de Coubertin. It's based on the notion of a Napoleonic military messenger having to ride, fence, shoot, swim and run his way back to headquarters. According to the baron, it was meant to test a man's moral qualities as much as his physical resources and skills. Events in Seoul certainly tested Watson's moral fabric, and to the core, but hardly in the way he planned.

**John Coates (voiceover):** Early yesterday morning the IOC Medical Commission delivered to our room in the Village notification that the first urine sample from Alex was positive. Alex informed the IOC that he had consumed 10 to 12 cups of coffee, which he had obtained at the venue on the day. I have been told that to record such a high level of caffeine from a normal consumption of coffee would render one violently ill and unable to participate in the competition.

**Alex Watson (voiceover):** I must say firstly that I am entirely innocent. I have never taken drugs, other than whatever caffeine there is in coffee and Coca-Cola, and I took no prohibited drugs in Seoul.

**Warwick Hadfield:** Alex Watson at a press conference after being sent home from Seoul. And before him, John Coates, the Chef de Mission of the Australian team in 1988 and now Australia's most senior Olympic official. I was at that announcement in Seoul, and I remember well the disbelief that filled the room. As a result of the positive sample taken during the fencing part of the Pentathlon, the IOC disqualified Watson from the Olympics. The International Pentathlon body imposed a two-year ban on him, and an embarrassed and

Transcript from Sports Factor: ABC Radio National, February 6 2004.

irritated Australian Olympic Federation banned him for life. That meant he could never represent his country again. It all came as an unholy shock for Watson, who was not just a capable athlete, but a respected promoter of the Olympic movement here in Australia.

**Alex Watson:** It was kind of an unreal feeling. It was like I was going to pinch myself and wake up, and this would all have been a bad nightmare. And 10 o'clock that morning, as we were flying out, forced to fly out, that's, you know the run was starting in which I should have been a strong contender for a medal. So the whole thing had a real feeling of unreality about it, and because I was really just as confused as the AOC as to what possibly could have happened. And I guess in their shoes, I can't blame them for the actions they took at the time.

**Warwick Hadfield:** You got on the aeroplane, and you're obviously feeling this air of unreality, but between Seoul and Hong Kong, reality must have hit you, because you then got to Hong Kong and turned around and came back to Seoul and went back into the Village to talk to those officials again.

**Alex Watson:** I knew in my heart that I had done nothing wrong. So I knew that I was being unfairly dismissed from competition, and there's got to be some explanation. What it was, I wasn't sure. I felt someone could have spiked my drinks, that seemed a reasonable possibility, but I was really angry and confused and very angry about the fact that having a good strong competition with a chance to win Australia's first medal in this sport, that I was being taken out of the game.

**Warwick Hadfield:** And you came back, and you suggested that someone might have spiked your drink; what was the reaction to that from the Olympic officials then, people like John Coates and the rest of the team?

**Alex Watson:** Oh well, they were furious.

**Warwick Hadfield:** With you?

**Alex Watson:** Yes.

**Warwick Hadfield:** They didn't want you there.

**Alex Watson:** Well as far as they were concerned, at this stage I'd done the wrong thing, I'd tried to cheat, I'd failed a drug test, I was a disgrace, and they didn't want to hear from me, they wanted to concentrate on athletes who were still in competition and rightly so.

**Warwick Hadfield:** And how did you feel about that?

**Alex Watson:** I was really hoping that right up until when I was kicked out that the phone was going to ring and someone from the IOC laboratory was going to go, 'Oops, sorry, we got the wrong sample.'

**Warwick Hadfield:** Now you eventually did come home to Australia. What was the reaction when you got off the aeroplane in this country, given that you were by now labelled very much a drug cheat?

**Alex Watson:** Well I was met by a gentleman from the Federal Airports Corporation who—there'd been a press conference set up at the airport, and I remember getting off the plane, and he said to me, 'Have you ever done a press conference?' and I said, 'Oh, I've done some media interviews and things.' And he said, 'Well I hope you're ready for this, because there's a room jam-packed with all of Australia's media.' So it was pretty daunting.

**Warwick Hadfield:** And did you get the grill? I mean obviously when you're in the public spotlight like that, and the media turns out, did you feel the intensity of their questions?

**Alex Watson:** I felt that everyone was really looking at me eyeball-to-eyeball, just trying to get a gauge of 'Look, is this guy on the level or is he telling us lies?'

**Warwick Hadfield:** When did you make up your mind not to accept what was then a life ban, and what processes did you put in place then?

**Alex Watson:** Well I never accepted that I should have a life ban, or any ban, because as I said, I knew in my heart that I had not tried to cheat, and anything that had happened, had to be an accident or a mistake, and so right from the word go I was fighting it. But really, the breakthrough came when Professor Don Birkett, from Flinders University, came out publicly of his own accord and basically contacted *The Australian* newspaper and said, 'Look, I'm reading all this stuff, I don't have any real interest or background in sport, I'm a scientist. But I can tell you everything the AOC and the IOC Medical Commission are saying about what this guy must have done to breach the caffeine test is a load of nonsense, and I can prove it to you.'

**Warwick Hadfield:** Birkett and his colleague, Dr. John Miner, were able to do just that. Through Miner's wife, a fencer, they were aware of the culture of coffee drinking in that sport during competition. And through their own research they knew that a reading like the one Watson recorded in Seoul, 14 milligrams per litre, could in some people, be reached by drinking as little as three or four cups of coffee. Suddenly the tide of public opinion turned away from the Olympic movement and in favour of Watson.

**Kevan Gosper (IOC official and Australian Olympic Committee Board Member) (voiceover):** Having considered all the matters, the Board considers that Alex Watson's disqualification by the International Olympic Committee in Seoul was in itself severe punishment. Since then, the necessary drawn-out processes added to the personal anguish that he's clearly suffered. Accordingly, today we decided not to apply a life ban, which leaves Alex Watson to be considered for selection in future Australian Olympic teams.

**Warwick Hadfield:** His life suspension reduced to two years by Australian Olympic officials, and the criticism of those officials by a Federal Parliamentary Inquiry into Drugs in Sport, did much to restore Watson's reputation. But it wasn't without its costs. At times he became both angry and depressed, as he fought to clear his name. And despite the assistance of an uncle who was a highly qualified lawyer, his legal bills still reached six figures. All up, it was an expensive lesson in life.

**Alex Watson:** The thing I think that really helped me was being a sportsperson because when I got really depressed, what I did was, I went out and I ran, or I rode my horses, or I actually went to swimming training. My people in my swim squad stood by me. Some people were absolutely marvellous, they just carried on and supported me as though it had never happened, and so I had a close circle of friends and I tried to just lead a normal life. And the thing that really helped was also going out into places, the local shops. I went into a supermarket a couple of days after I was home, to get some groceries, and people just came up to me in the supermarket and said, 'We know you didn't do it. Fight the bastards.' And I never had one person in public ridicule me or come up and verbally abuse me or anything. So that gave me a great feeling of support.

**Warwick Hadfield:** 'Drug cheat'; that's a stigma that sticks. When do you think people are going to say, 'Alex Watson' without thinking of the rest of that, 'drug cheat'; 'sent home from Seoul'. Will that ever happen, or will that always be part of your life now?

**Alex Watson:** Well I don't think you can ever escape being the Cappuccino Kid, it's a nickname that's probably going to stick with me forever. But it's turned around into really largely a positive.

**Warwick Hadfield:** Testing positive, to turning into a positive.

**Alex Watson:** Yes. I mean it is. I mean I have—after it all was cleared up. The only thing it's on the records still that I failed a test and was sent home from the Games. But I turned it around and went back and made the Olympic team in '92.

**Warwick Hadfield:** On January 1st this year, the new World Anti-Doping Authority, WADA, released its first list of prohibited substances. Missing was caffeine. I asked the head of the Australian Sports Drug Agency, John Mendoza, if this was an admission there were flaws in the Watson case.

**John Mendoza (voiceover):** It's more an admission or a recognition that caffeine is used in many societies as part of the standard sort of food and beverage consumption, and in fact what we now know about caffeine, which we didn't know in 1988, is that the performance enhancement effect is actually best, if you like, there's a mild stimulant effect, but the effect is a positive one when it's about half what the actual banned level was. And if we were to take it down to a 6-nanogram-per-ml level, it would simply mean that athletes could not consume caffeine products and that's a very wide range of products, not just coffee, in their day-to-day lives. Now that is unrealistic, and it's unnecessary because the effect is a very mild stimulant effect. So commonsense I think prevailed there, and we've seen caffeine removed from the list.

**Warwick Hadfield:** Both John Mendoza and John Coates say Watson's disqualification will never be overturned by the IOC even though many now believe it was unjust. They argue that the offence occurred under the rules of the time. But Alex Watson hasn't given up hope entirely.

**Alex Watson:** I'd like to see that happen. I mean let's face it, if that happened, that's also a plus for the AOC, because it means one of their athletes who was supposedly kicked out of the Games, found guilty, wasn't. So it's a plus for Australian sport too. But I think John is alluding to the fact that reading between the lines, as he knows as well as I do, he's now an IOC member, just how difficult it is to take the IOC on. It's virtually impossible. I mean we tried to take them to the Court of Arbitration for Sport in The Hague, the court that they set up. But the rules of the Court of Arbitration for Sport are that both parties must agree to have the matter heard. We were agreed, but they wouldn't agree to go to their own court, because they know their legal people told them, 'Look, if this guy proves his case, you threw him out of the Olympic Games. You're leaving yourself wide open', and that's exactly why they won't play ball. I mean the Parliamentary Committee into Drugs in Sport highlighted this aspect and said the IOC have failed their own test of integrity. But the fact is, when they pull the shutters down and won't play ball, they're bloody impossible to deal with because you can't pin them in any country, you've got to rely on their co-operation.

**Warwick Hadfield:** Alex, is this the end of it all, and I presume in 2004 you've come to grips with it as best as you're ever going to. If someone said to you, 'How do you feel about the whole incident now?,' how do you sum it up?

**Alex Watson:** I'd sum it up as a life-changing experience, because it taught me to not believe everything you hear and see, and not judge everything on first case; look behind the scenes and also it taught me the value of family and true friends, because, to put it bluntly, when the shit hits the fan, it's the people who stick by you, they're the people that really count. There's lots of back-slappers and lots of well-wishers when you're on top of the world. When I won the show-jumping on Day 1 in Seoul, I had people saying, 'Oh, won't it be great when you win the gold medal and your life will change, and what a great guy you are', and when the shit hit the fan two days or three days later, there weren't many of them around.

# References and Reading List

## Chapter 1 A Brief History of Caffeine in Sport

Arctander, S. 1960. Cola. In *Perfume and flavor materials of natural origin*, ed. S. Arctander, pp. 187-188. Elizabeth, NJ: Steffen Arctander.

Asmussen, E., and Boje, O. 1947. The effect of alcohol and some drugs on the capacity for work. *Acta Physiol Scand* 15:109-113.

Blumenthal, M. 2000. Cola nut. In *Herbal medicine: Expanded commission e reviews*, eds. A. Goldberg, M. Blumenthal, S. Foster, and J. Brinckmann, pp. 72-73. Newton, MA: Integrative Medicine Communications.

Foltz, E., Ivy, A., and Barborka, C. 1943. The influence of amphetamine (benzedrine) sulfate, d-desoxyephedrinehydrochloride (pervitin), and caffeine upon work output and recovery when rapidly exhausting work is done by trained subjects. *J Lab Clin Med* 28:603-606.

Foltz, E., Schiffrin, M., and Ivy, A. 1943. The influence of amphetamine (benzedrine) sulfate and caffeine on the performance of rapidly exhausting work by untrained subjects. *J Lab Clin Med* 28:601-603.

Haldi, J., and Wynn, W. 1946. Action of drugs on efficiency of swimmers. *Research Quart* 17:96-101.

Hoberman, J. 2013. Dopers on wheels: The Tour's sorry history. NBC Sports. http://nbcsports.msnbc.com/id/19462071/ns/sports-tour_de_france/

Murray, T. 1983. The coercive power of drugs in sports. *Hastings Center Report* 13(4): 24-30.

Rivers, W., and Webber, H. 1907. The action of caffeine on the capacity for muscular work. *J Physiol* 36:33-47.

## Chapter 2 How Caffeine Works

Birkett, D.J., and Miners, J.O. 1991. Caffeine renal clearance and urine caffeine concentrations during steady-state dosing: Implications for monitoring caffeine intake during sports events. *Brit J Clin Pharmacol* 31:405-408.

Chesley, A., Howlett, R.A., Heigenhauser, G.J.F., Hultman, E., and Spriet, LL. 1996. Regulation of muscle glycogen phosphorylase activity during intense aerobic exercise following caffeine ingestion. *Am J Physiol* 275:R596-R603.

Costill, D.L., Dalsky, G.P., and Fink, W.J. 1978. Effects of caffeine on metabolism and exercise performance. *Med Sci Sports* 10:155-158.

Cox, G.R., Desbrow, B., Montgomery, P.G., Anderson, M.E., Bruce, C.R., Macrides, T.A., Martin, D.T., Moquin, A., Roberts, A., Hawley, J.A., and Burke, L.M. 2002. Effect of different protocols of caffeine intake on metabolism and endurance performance. *J Appl Physiol* 93:990-999.

Daly, J.W. 1993. Mechanism of action of caffeine. In *Caffeine, coffee, and health*, ed. S. Garattini, pp. 97-150. New York: Raven Press.

Davis, J.M., and Bailey, S.P. 1997. Possible mechanisms of central nervous system fatigue during exercise. *Med Sci Sports Exerc* 29:45-57.

Davis, J.M., Zhao, Z., Stock, H.S., Mehl, K.A., Buggy, J., and Hand, G.A. 2003. Central nervous system effects of caffeine and adenosine on fatigue. *Am J Physiol* 284:R399-R404.

Desbrow, B., Barrett, C.M., Minahan, C.L., Grant, G.D., and Leveritt, M.D. 2009. Caffeine, cycling performance, and exogenous CHO oxidation: A dose–response study. *Med Sci Sports Exerc* 41:1744-1751.

Fernstrom, J.D., and Fernstrom, M.H. 1984. Effects of caffeine on monamine neurotransmitters in the central and peripheral nervous system. In *Caffeine*, ed. P.B. Dews, pp. 107-118. Berlin: Springer-Verlag.

Fredholm, B.B. 1995. Adenosine, adenosine receptors and the actions of caffeine. *Pharm Tox* 76:93-101.

Graham, T.E., and Spriet, L.L. 1991. Performance and metabolic responses to a high caffeine dose during prolonged exercise. *J Appl Physiol* 71:2292-2298.

Graham, T.E., and Spriet, L.L. 1995. Metabolic, catecholamine, and exercise performance: responses to various doses of caffeine. *J Appl Physiol* 78:867-874.

Graham, T.E., Helge, J.W., MacLean, D.A., Kiens, B., and Richter, E.A. 2000. Caffeine ingestion does not alter carbohydrate or fat metabolism in skeletal muscle during exercise. *J Physiol* 529(3): 837-847.

Hetzler, R.K., Knowlton, R.G., Somani, S.M., Brown, D.D., and Perkins, R.M. 1990. Effect of paraxanthine on FFA mobilization after intravenous caffeine administration in humans. *J Appl Physiol* 68:44-47.

Hulston, C.J., and Jeukendrup, A.E. 2008. Substrate metabolism and exercise performance with caffeine and carbohydrate intake. *Med Sci Sports Exerc* 40:2096-2104.

Jentjens, R.L., Venables, M.C., and Jeukendrup, A. 2004. Oxidation of exogenous glucose, sucrose and maltose during prolonged cycling exercise. *J Appl Physiol* 96:1285-1291.

Kalmar, J.M., and Cafarelli, E. 2004. Caffeine: A valuable tool to study central fatigue in humans. *Exerc Sports Sci Rev* 32:143-147.

Lindinger, M.I., Graham, T.E., and Spriet, L.L. 1993. Caffeine attenuates the exercise-induced increase in plasma [$K^+$] in humans. *J Appl Physiol* 74:1149-1155.

Nehlig, A., Daval, J.-L., and Debry, G. 1992. Caffeine and the central nervous system: mechanisms of action, biochemical, metabolic, and psychostimulant effects. *Brain Res Rev* 17:139-170.

Nehlig, A., and Debry, G. 1994. Caffeine and sports activity: a review. *Int J Sports Med* 15:215-223.

Spriet, L.L. 2003. Caffeine. In *Performance-enhancing substances in sport and exercise*, eds. M.S. Bahrke and C.E. Yesalis (pp. 267-278). Windsor, ON: Human Kinetics.

Spriet, L.L., and Howlett, R.A. 2000. Caffeine. In *Nutrition in sport—encyclopaedia of sports medicine*, ed. R.J. Maughan (Vol. VII, pp. 379-392). Oxford: Blackwell Science.

Spriet, L.L., MacLean, D.A., Dyck, D.J., Hultman, E., Cederblad, G., and Graham, T.E. 1992. Caffeine ingestion and muscle metabolism during prolonged exercise in humans. *Am J Physiol* 262:E891-E898.

Talanian, J.L., and Spriet, L.L. 2007. Low doses of caffeine late in exercise improve cycling time trial performance. *FASEB J* 21:107 (abstract).

Wallace, S. 2012. Players' use of caffeine to boost performance is ridiculous, claims expert. *The Independent*. www.independent.co.uk/sport/football/international/players-use-of-caffeine-pills-to-boost-performance-is-ridiculous-claims-expert-8217239.html.

Yeo, S.E., Jentjens, R.L.P.G., Wallis, G.A., and Jeukendrup, A.E. 2005. Caffeine increases exogenous carbohydrate oxidation during exercise. *J Appl Physiol* 99:844-850.

# Chapter 3 Finding Caffeine in Our Diets

Buxton, C., and Hagan, J.E. 2012. A survey of energy drinks consumption practices among student-athletes in Ghana: Lessons for developing health education intervention programmes. *J Int Soc Sports Nutr* 9(1): 9.

Chou, K.-H., and Bell, L. 2007. Caffeine content of prepackaged national-brand and private-label carbonated beverages. *J Food Sci* 72(6): C337-C342.

Consumer Reports. 2012. The buzz on energy-drink caffeine. www.consumerreports.org/cro/magazine/2012/12/the-buzz-on-energy-drink-caffeine/index.htm. Accessed January 13, 2013.

Desbrow, B., Hughes, R., Leveritt, M., and Scheelings, P. 2007. An independent analysis of consumer exposure to caffeine from retail coffees. *Food Chem Toxicol* 45:1588-1592.

Food Standards Agency (FSA). 2004. Survey of caffeine levels in hot beverages. Food Survey Information Sheet 53/04.

Keast, R., and Riddell, L. 2007. Caffeine as a flavor additive in soft-drinks. *Appetite* 49:255-259.

McCusker, R.R., Goldberger, B.A., and Cone, E.J. 2003. Caffeine content of specialty coffees. *J Anal Toxicol* 27:520-522.

Panek, L.M., Swoboda, C., Bendlin, A., and Temple, J.L. 2013. Caffeine increases liking and consumption of novel-flavored yogurt. *Psychopharmacology* (Berl). [Epub ahead of print]

# Chapter 4 Caffeine Use in Daily Life

American Psychiatric Association (APA). 2000. *Diagnostic and statistical manual of mental disorders: DSM-IV-TR*. Washington, DC: Author.

Boos, C.J., Simms, P., Morris, F.R., and Fertout, M. 2011. The use of exercise and dietary supplements among British soldiers in Afghanistan. *J R Army Med Corps* 157(3): 229-232.

Buxton, C., and Hagan, J.E. 2012. A survey of energy drinks consumption practices among student-athletes in Ghana: Lessons for developing health education intervention programmes. *J Int Soc Sports Nutr* 9(1): 9.

Centers for Disease Control and Prevention (CDC). 2012. Energy drink consumption and its association with sleep problems among U.S. service members on a combat deployment - Afghanistan, 2010. MMWR *Morb Mortal Wkly Rep.* 61(44):895-8.

Chester, N., and Wojek, N. 2008 Caffeine consumption amongst British athletes following changes to the 2004 WADA prohibited list. *Int J Sports Med* 29:524-528.

Del Coso, J., Muñoz, G., and Muñoz-Guerra, J. 2011. Prevalence of caffeine use in elite athletes following its removal from the World Anti-Doping Agency list of banned substances. *Appl Physiol Nutr Metab* 36:555-561.

Dascombe, B., Karunaratna, M., Cartoon, J., Fergie, B., and Goodman, C. 2010. Nutritional supplementation habits and perceptions of elite athletes within a state-based sporting institute. *J Sci Med Sport* 13(2): 274-280.

Froiland, K., Koszewski, W., Hingst, J., and Kopecky, L. 2004. Nutritional supplement use among college athletes and their sources of information. *Int J Sport Nut Ex Metab* 14:104-120.

Hoyte, C.O., Albert, D., and Heard, K.J. 2013. The use of energy drinks, dietary supplements, and prescription medications by United States college students to enhance athletic performance. *J Community Health* [Epub ahead of print]

Ker, K., Edwards, P.J., Felix, L.M., Blackhall, K., and Roberts, I. 2010. Caffeine for the prevention of injuries and errors in shift workers. The Cochrane Library. Published online: May 12. http://onlinelibrary.wiley.com/doi/10.1002/14651858.CD008508/abstract

Kristiansen, M., Levy-Milne, R., Barr, S., and Flint, A. 2005. Dietary supplement use by varsity athletes at a Canadian university. *Int J Sport Nut Ex Metab* 15:195-210.

Lieberman, H.R., Stavinoha, T.B., McGraw, S.M., White, A., Hadden, L.S., and Marriott, B.P. 2010. Use of dietary supplements among active-duty US Army soldiers. *Am J Clin Nutr* 92(4): 985-995.

Malinauskas, B.M., Aeby, V.G., Overton, R.F., Carpenter-Aeby, T., and Barber-Heidal, K. 2007. A survey of energy drink consumption patterns among college students. *Nutr J* 31:35.

Mets, M.A.J., Baas, D., van Boven, I., Olivier, B., and Verster, J.C. 2012. Effects of coffee on driving performance during prolonged simulated highway driving. *Psychopharmacology* 222:337-342.

Slater, G., Tan, B., and Teh, K.C. 2003. Dietary supplementation practices of Singaporean athletes. *Int J Sport Nut Ex Metab* 13(3): 320-332.

Vail, V. 2012. Q&A with Chris McCormack. http://vivienvail.com/2012/06/28/qa-with-chris-mccormack.

Van Thuyne, W., and Delbeke, F.T. 2006. Distribution of caffeine levels in urine in different sports in relation to doping control before and after the removal of caffeine from the WADA doping list. *Int J Sports Med* 27(9): 745-750

Van Thuyne, W., Roels, K., and Delbeke, F.T. 2005. Distribution of caffeine levels in urine in different sports in relation to doping control. *Int J Sports Med* 26(9): 714-718.

# Chapter 5 Effectiveness

Acker-Hewitt, T.L., Shafer, B.M., Saunders, M.J., Goh, Q., Luden, N.D. 2012. Independent and combined effects of carbohydrate and caffeine ingestion on aerobic cycling performance in the fed state. *Appl Physiol Nutr Metab* 37:276-283.

Anderson, M.E., Bruce, C.R., Fraser, S.F., Stepto, N.K., Klein, R., Hopkins, W.G., and Hawley, J.A. 2000. Improved 2000-meter rowing performance in competitive oarswomen after caffeine ingestion. *Int J Sport Nutr Exerc Metab* 10:464-475.

Astorino, T.A., Cottrell, T., Lozano, A.T., Aburto-Pratt, K., and Duhon, J. 2012a. Acute caffeine ingestion's increase of voluntarily chosen resistance-training load after limited sleep. *Nutr Res* 32(2): 78-84.

Astorino, T.A., Cottrell, T., Talhami Lozano, A., Aburto-Pratt, K., and Duhon, J. 2012b. Effect of caffeine on RPE and perceptions of pain, arousal, and pleasure/displeasure during a cycling time trial in endurance trained and active men. *Physiol Behav* 106(2): 211-217.

Astorino TA, Matera AJ, Basinger J, Evans M, Schurman T, Marquez R. 2012c. Effects of red bull energy drink on repeated sprint performance in women athletes. *Amino Acids* 42(5):1803-8.

Astorino, T.A., and Roberson, D.W. 2010. Efficacy of acute caffeine ingestion for short-term high-intensity exercise performance: a systematic review. *J Strength Cond Res.* 24(1):257-65

Astorino, T.A., Rohmann, R.L., and Firth K. 2008. Effect of caffeine ingestion on one-repetition maximum muscular strength. *Eur J Appl Physiol* 102:127-132.

Bassini, A., Magalhães-Neto, A.M., Sweet, E., Bottino, A., Veiga, C., Tozzi, M.B., Pickard, M.B. and Cameron, L.C. 2013. Caffeine decreases systemic urea in elite soccer players during intermittent exercise. *Med Sci Sports Exerc.* 45(4):683-690.

Batterham, A.M., and Hopkins, W.G. 2006. Making meaningful inferences about magnitudes. *Int J Sports Physiol Perform* 1:50-57.

Beaven, C. M., Maulder, P., Poolev, A., Kilduff, L., and Cook, C. 2013. Effects of caffeine and carbohydrate mouth rinses on repeated sprint performance. *Appl Physiol Nutr Metab* 38:633-637.

Beck, T.W., Housh, T.J., Malek, M.H., Mielke, M. and Hendrix, R. 2008. The acute effects of a caffeine-containing supplement on bench press strength and time to running exhaustion. *J Strength Cond Res.*22(5):1654-8.

Beedie, C.J., Stuart, E.M., Coleman, D.A., and Foad, A.J. 2006. Placebo effects of caffeine on cycling performance. *Med Sci Sports Exerc* 38:2159-2164.

Bell, D.G., and McLellan, T.M. 2002. Exercise endurance 1, 3, and 6 h after caffeine ingestion in caffeine users and nonusers. *J Appl Physiol* 93:1227-1234.

Bell, D.G., and McLellan, T.M. 2003. Effect of repeated caffeine ingestion on repeated exhaustive exercise endurance. *Med Sci Sports Exerc* 35:1348-1354.

Bellar, D.M., Kamimori, G., Judge, L., Barkley, J.E., Ryan, E.J., Muller, M., and Glickman, E.L. 2012. Effects of low-dose caffeine supplementation on early morning performance in the standing shot put throw. *Eur J Sports Sci* 12(1): 57-61.

Berglund, B., and Hemmingsson, P. 1982. Effects of caffeine ingestion on exercise performance at low and high altitudes in cross-country skiers. *Int J Sports Med* 3:234-236.

Bottoms, L., Greenhalgh, A., and Gregory, K. 2013. The effect of caffeine ingestion on skill maintenance and fatigue in epee fencers. *J Sports Sci.*[Epub ahead of print]

Bridge, C.A., and Jones, M.A. 2006. The effect of caffeine ingestion on 8 km run performance in a field setting. *J Sports Sci* 24:433-439.

Bruce, C.R., Anderson, M.E., Fraser, S.F., Stepto, N.K., Klein, R., Hopkins, W.G., and Hawley, J.A. 2000. Enhancement of 2000-m rowing performance after caffeine ingestion. *Med Sci Sports Exerc* 32:1958-1963.

Carpenter, M. 2012. Caffeine gives endurance athletes a third and fourth wind. *NPR News.* http://m.npr.org/news/Health/165157480.

Carr, A., Dawson, B., Schneiker, K., Goodman, C., and Lay, B. 2008. Effect of caffeine supplementation on repeated sprint running performance. *J Sports Med Phys Fitness* 48:472-478.

Carr, A.J., Gore, C.J., and Dawson, B. 2011. Induced alkalosis and caffeine supplementation: effects on 2,000-m rowing performance. *Int J Sport Nutr Exerc Metab* 21:357-364.

Cohen, B.S., Nelson, A.G., Prevost, M.C., Thompson, G.D., Marx, B.D., and Morris, G.S. 1996. Effects of caffeine ingestion on endurance racing in heat and humidity. *Eur J Appl Physiol* 73:358-363.

Collomp, K., Ahmaidi, S., Chatard, J.C., Audran, M., and Prefaut, C. 1992. Benefits of caffeine ingestion on sprint performance in trained and untrained swimmers. *Eur J Appl Physiol* 64:377-380.

Conger, S.A., Warren, G.L., Hardy, M.A., and Millard-Stafford, M.L. 2011. Does caffeine added to carbohydrate provide additional ergogenic benefit for endurance? *Int J Sport Nutr Exerc Metab* 21:71-84.

Conway, K.J., Orr, R., and Stannard, S.R. 2003. Effect of a divided dose of endurance cycling performance, postexercise urinary caffeine concentration and plasma paraxanthine. *J Appl Physiol* 94:1557-1562.

Cook, C., Beaven, C.M., Kilduff, L.P., and Drawer, S. 2012. Acute caffeine ingestion's increase of voluntarily chosen resistance-training load after limited sleep. *Int J Sport Nutr Exerc Metab* 22(3): 157-164.

Cox, G.R., Desbrow, B., Montgomery, P.G., Anderson, M.E., Bruce, C.R., Macrides, T.A., Martin, D.T., Moquin, A., Roberts, A., Hawley, J.A., and Burke, L.M. 2002. Effect of different protocols of caffeine intake on metabolism and endurance performance. *J Appl Physiol* 93:990-999.

Crawford, S. 2010. Caffeine critics need to take a chill pill. *Sunday Herald Sun.* www.heraldsun.com.au/afl/more-news/caffeine-critics-need-to-take-a-chill-pill/story-e6frf9jf-1225890284314

Cureton, K.J., Warren, G.L., Millard-Stafford, M.L., Wingo, J.E., Trilk, J., and Buyckx, M. 2007. Caffeinated sports drink: ergogenic effects and possible mechanisms. *Int J Sport Nutr Exerc Metab* 17:35-55.

Del Coso, J., Portillo, J., Muñoz, G., Abián-Vicén, J., Gonzalez-Millán, C., and Muñoz-Guerra, J. 2013. Caffeine-containing energy drink improves sprint performance during an international rugby sevens competition. *Amino Acids.* [Epub ahead of print]

Del Coso, J., Muñoz-Fernández, V.E., Muñoz, G., Fernández-Elías, V.E., Ortega, J.F., Hamouti, N., Barbero, J.C., and Muñoz-Guerra, J. 2012a. Effects of a caffeine-containing energy drink on simulated soccer performance. *PLoS One* 7(2).

Del Coso, J., Salinero, J.J., González-Millán, C., Abián-Vicén, J., and Pérez-González, B. 2012b. Dose–response effects of a caffeine-containing energy drink on muscle performance: a repeated measures design. *J Int Soc Sports Nutr* 9(1): 21.

Desbrow, B., Barrett, C.M., Minahan, C.L., Grant, G.D., and Leveritt, M.D. 2009. Caffeine, cycling performance, and exogenous CHO oxidation: a dose–response study. *Med Sci Sports Exerc* 41:1744-1751.

Desbrow, B., Biddulph, C., Devlin, B., Grant, G.D., Anoopkumar-Dukie, S., and Leveritt, M.D. 2012. The effects of different doses of caffeine on endurance cycling time trial performance. *J Sports Sci* 30:115-120.

Desbrow, B., and Leveritt, M. 2006. Awareness and use of caffeine by athletes competing at the 2005 Ironman Triathlon World Championships. *Int J Sport Nutr Exerc Metab* 16:545-558.

Doherty, M., and Smith, P.M. 2004. Effects of caffeine ingestion on exercise testing. *Int J Sport Nutr Exerc Metab* 14:626-646.

Duncan, M.J., and Oxford, S.W. 2011. The effect of caffeine ingestion on mood state and bench press performance to failure. *J Strength Cond Res* 25:178-185.

Duncan, M.J., Smith, M., Cook, K., and James, R.S. 2012. The acute effect of a caffeine-containing energy drink on mood state, readiness to invest effort, and resistance exercise to failure. *J Strength Cond Res* 26(10): 2858-2865.

Duncan, M.J., Taylor, S., and Lyons, M. 2012. The effect of caffeine ingestion on field hockey skill performance following physical fatigue. *Res Sports Med* 20(1): 25-36.

Duvnjak-Zaknich, D.M., Dawson, B.T., Wallman, K.E., and Henry, G. 2011. Effect of caffeine on reactive agility time when fresh and fatigued. *Med Sci Sports Exerc* 43:1523-1530.

Eckerson, J.M., Bull, A.J., Baechle, T.R., Fischer, C.A., O'Brien, D.C., Moore, G.A., Yee, J.C., and Pulverenti, T.S. 2012. Acute ingestion of sugar-free Red Bull energy drink has no effect on upper body strength and muscular endurance in resistance trained men. *J Strength Cond Res*. E-pub ahead of print.

Ferrauti, A., Weber, K., and Struder, H.K. 1997. Metabolic and ergogenic effects of carbohydrate and caffeine beverages in tennis. *J Sports Med Phys Fitness* 37:258-266.

Fiala, K.A., Casa, D.J., and Roti, M.W. 2004. Rehydration with a caffeinated beverage during the nonexercise periods of 3 consecutive days of 2-a-day practices. *Int J Sport Nutr Exerc Metab* 14:419-429.

Foad, A.J., Beedie, C.J., and Coleman, D.A. 2008. Pharmacological and psychological effects of caffeine ingestion in 40-km cycling performance. *Med Sci Sports Exerc* 40(1): 158-165.

Foskett, A., Ali, A., and Gant, N. 2009. Caffeine enhances cognitive function and skill performance during simulated soccer activity. *Int J Sport Nutr Exerc Metab*.9(4): 410-423

Ganio, M.S., Johnson, E.C., Klau, J.F., Anderson, J.M., Casa, D.J., Maresh, C.M., Volek, J.S., and Armstrong, L.E. 2011. Effect of ambient temperature on caffeine ergogenicity during endurance exercise. *Eur J Appl Physiol* 111:1135-1146.

Ganio, M.S., Klau, J.F., Lee, E.C., Yeargin, S.W., McDermott, B.P., Buyckx, M., Maresh, C.M., and Armstrong, L.E. 2010. Effect of various carbohydrate-electrolyte fluids on cycling performance and maximal voluntary contraction. *Int J Sport Nutr Exerc Metab* 20:104-114.

Gant, N., Ali, A., and Foskett, A. 2010. The influence of caffeine and carbohydrate coingestion on simulated soccer performance. *Int J Sport Nutr Exerc Metab* 20:191-197.

Glaister, M., Howatson, G., Abraham, C.S., Lockey, R.A., Goodwin, J.E., Foley, P., and McInnes, G. 2008. Caffeine supplementation and multiple sprint running performance. *Med Sci Sports Exerc* 40:1835-1840.

Glaister, M., Patterson, S.D., Foley, P., Pedlar, C.R., Pattison, J.R., and McInnes, G. 2012. Caffeine and sprinting performance: dose responses and efficacy. *J Strength Cond Res* 26:1001-1005.

Goldstein, E., Jacobs, P.L., Whitehurst, M., Penhollow, T., and Antonio, J. 2010. Caffeine enhances upper body strength in resistance-trained women. *J Int Soc Sports Nutr* 7:18.

Goldstein, E.R., Ziegenfuss, T., Kalman, D., Kreider, R., Campbell, B., Wilborn, C., Taylor, L., Willoughby, D., Stout, J., Graves, B.S., Wildman, R., Ivy, J.L., Spano, M., Smith, A.E., and Antonio, J. 2010. International Society of Sports Nutrition position stand: caffeine and performance. *J Int Soc Sports Nutr* 7(1): 5.

Gonzalez-Alonso J., Heaps, C.L., and Coyle, E.F. 1992. Rehydration after exercise with common beverages and water. *Int J Sports Med* 13:399-406.

Graham, T.E. 2001a. Caffeine, coffee and ephedrine: impact on exercise performance and metabolism. *Can J Appl Physiol* 26:S103-S109.

Graham, T.E. 2001b. Caffeine and exercise: metabolism, endurance and performance. *Sports Med* 31:765-785.

Graham, T.E., Battram, D.S., Dela, F., El-Sohemy, A., and Thong, F.S. 2008. Does caffeine alter muscle carbohydrate and fat metabolism during exercise? *Appl Physiol Nutr Metab* 33:1311-1318.

Graham, T.E., Hibbert, E., and Sathasivam, P. 1998. Metabolic and exercise endurance effects of coffee and caffeine ingestion. *J Appl Physiol* 85: 883-889.

Graham, T.E., and Spriet, L.L. 1995. Metabolic, catecholamine, and exercise performance responses to various doses of caffeine. *J Appl Physiol* 78:867-874.

Gwacham, N., and Wagner, D.R. 2012. Acute effects of a caffeine-taurine energy drink on repeated sprint performance of American college football players. *Int J Sport Nutr Exerc Metab* 22:109-116.

Hodgson, A.B., Randell, R.K., and Jeukendrup, A.E. 2013. The metabolic and performance effects of caffeine compared to coffee during endurance exercise. *PLoS ONE* 8(4): e59561.

Hopkins, W.G., Hawley, J.A., and Burke, L.M. 1999. Design and analysis of research on sport performance enhancement. *Med Sci Sports Exerc* 31:472-485.

Hornery, D.J., Farrow, D., Mujika, I, and Young, W.B. 2007. Caffeine, carbohydrate, and cooling use during prolonged simulated tennis. *Int J Sports Physiol Perform.* 2(4):423-38

Hunter, A.M., St. Clair Gibson, A., Collins, M., Lambert, M., and Noakes, T.D. 2002. Caffeine ingestion does not alter performance during a 100-km cycling time-trial performance. *Int J Sport Nutr Exerc Metab* 12:438-452.

Irwin, C., Desbrow, B., Ellis, A., O'Keeffe, B., Grant, G., and Leveritt, M. 2011. Caffeine withdrawal and high-intensity endurance cycling performance. *J Sports Sci* 29:509-515.

Ivy, J.L., Kammer, L., Ding, Z., Wang., B, Bernard, J.R., Liao, Y.H., and Hwang, J. 2009. Improved cycling time-trial performance after ingestion of a caffeine energy drink. *Int J Sport Nutr Exerc Metab.* 19(1):61-78.

Ivy, J.L., Costill, D.L., Fink, W.J., and Lower, R.W. 1979. Influence of caffeine and carbohydrate feedings on endurance performance. *Med Sci Sports Exerc* 11:6-11.

Jacobson, T.L., Febbraio, M.A., Arkinstall, M.J., and Hawley, J.A. 2001. Effect of caffeine co-ingested with carbohydrate or fat on metabolism and performance in endurance-trained men. *Exp Physiol* 86:137-144.

Jenkins, N.T., Trilk, J.L., Singhal, A., O'Connor, P.J., and Cureton, K.J. 2008. Ergogenic effects of low doses of caffeine on cycling performance. *Int J Sports Nutr Exerc Metab* 18:328-342.

Keisler, B.D., and Armsey, T.D. 2006. Caffeine as an ergogenic aid. *Curr Sports Med* 5:215-219.

Kilding, A.E., Overton, C., and Gleave, J. 2012. Effects of caffeine, sodium bicarbonate, and their combined ingestion on high-intensity cycling performance. *Int J Sport Nutr Exerc Metab* 22:175-183.

Klein, C.S., Clawson, A., Martin, M., Saunders, M.J., Flohr, J.A., Bechtel, M.K., Dunham, W., Hancock, H., and Womack, C.J. 2012 The effect of caffeine on performance in collegiate tennis players. *J Caff Res.* 2(3): 111-116.

Kovacs, E.M.R., Stegen, J.H.C.H., and Brouns, F. 1998. Effect of caffeinated drinks on substrate metabolism, caffeine excretion, and performance. *J Appl Physiol* 85:709-715.

Lane, S.C., Areta, J.L., Bird, S.R., Coffey, V.G., Burke, L.M., Desbrow, B., Karagounis, L.G.,and Hawley, J.A. 2013. Caffeine Ingestion and Cycling Power Output in a Low or Normal Muscle Glycogen State. *Med Sci Sports Exerc.* [Epub ahead of print]

Lassiter, D.G., Kammer, L., Burns, J., Ding, Z., Kim, H., Lee J., and Ivy, J.L. 2012. Effect of an energy drink on physical and cognitive performance in trained cyclists. *J Caff Res.* 2 (4) 167-175.

MacIntosh, B.R., and Wright, B.M. 1995. Caffeine ingestion and performance of a 1,500-metre swim. *Can J Appl Physiol* 20:168-177.

Millard-Stafford, M.L., Cureton, K.J., Wingo, J.E., Trilk, J., Warren, G.L., and Buyckx, M. 2007. Hydration during exercise in warm, humid conditions: effect of caffeinated sports drink. *Int J Sport Nutr Exerc Metab* 17:163-177.

Newman, P. 2009. Kevin Pietersen exclusive: I can forgive but I'll never forget how I was sacked as captain... *Daily Mail.* www.dailymail.co.uk/sport/cricket/article-1165144/KEVIN-PIETERSEN-EXCLUSIVE-I-forgive-Ill-forget-I-sacked-captain.html

O'Rourke, M.P., O'Brien, B.J., Knez, W.L., and Paton, C.D. 2008. Caffeine has a small effect on 5-km running performance of well-trained and recreational runners. *J Sci Med Sport* 11:231-233.

Pasman, W.J., van Baak, M.A., Jeukendrup, A.E., and de Haan, A. 1995. The effect of different dosages of caffeine on endurance performance time. *Int J Sports Med* 16:225-230.

Paton, C.D., Hopkins, W.G., and Vollebregt, L. 2001. Little effect of caffeine ingestion on repeated sprints in team-sport athletes. *Med Sci Sports Exerc* 33:822-825.

Paton, C.D., Lowe, T., and Irvine, A. 2010. Caffeinated chewing gum increases repeated sprint performance and augments increases in testosterone in competitive cyclists. *Eur J Appl Physiol* 110:1243-1250.

Pruscino, C.L., Ross, M.L., Gregory, J.R., Savage, B., and Flanagan, T.R. 2008. The effects of sodium bicarbonate, caffeine and their combination on repeated 200-m freestyle performance. *Int J Sport Nutr Exerc Metab* 18:116-130.

Roberts, S.P., Stokes, K.A., Trewartha, G., Doyle, J., Hogben, P., and Thompson, D. 2010. Effects of carbohydrate and caffeine ingestion on performance during a rugby union simulation protocol. *J Sports Sci* 28:833-842.

Roelands, B., Buyse, L., Pauwels, F., Delbeke, F., Deventer, K., and Meeusen, R. 2011. No effect of caffeine on exercise performance in high ambient temperature. *Eur J Appl Physiol* 111:3089-3095.

Ryan, E.J., Kim, C.H., Fickes, E.J., Williamson, M., Muller, M.D., Barkley, J.E., Gunstad, J., and Glickman, E.L. 2013. Caffeine gum and cycling performance: a timing study. *J Strength Cond Res* 27:259-264

Schneiker, K.T., Bishop, D., Dawson, B., and Hackett, L.P. 2006. Effects of caffeine on prolonged intermittent-sprint ability in team-sport athletes. *Med Sci Sports Exerc* 38:578-585.

Skinner, T.L., Jenkins, D.G., Coombes, J.S., Taaffe, D.R., and Leveritt, M.D. 2010. Dose response of caffeine on 2000-m rowing performance. *Med Sci Sports Exerc* 42: 571-576.

Skinner, T.L., Jenkins, D.G., Taaffe, D.R., Leveritt, M.D., and Coombes, J.S. 2013 Coinciding exercise with peak serum caffeine does not improve cycling performance. *J Sci Med Sport* 16:54-59.

Souissi, M., Abedelmalek, S., Chtourou, H., Atheymen, R., Hakim, A., and Sahnoun, Z. 2012. Effects of morning caffeine' ingestion on mood States, simple reaction time, and short-term maximal performance on elite judoists. *Asian J Sports Med.*3(3):161-8.

Spradley, B.D., Crowley, K.R., Tai, C.Y., Kendall, K.L., Fukuda, D.H., Esposito, E.N., Moon, S.E., and Moon, J.R. 2012. Ingesting a pre-workout supplement containing caffeine, B-vitamins, amino acids, creatine, and beta-alanine before exercise delays fatigue while improving reaction time and muscular endurance. *Nutr Metab (Lond)* 9:28.

Stadheim, H.K., Kvamme, B., Olsen, R. Drevon, C.A., Ivy, J.L., and Jensen, J. 2013. Caffeine increases performance in cross-1 country double poling time trial exercise. *Med Sci Sports Exerc.* [Epub ahead of print].

Stracher, C. 2013. *Kings of the road: How Frank Shorter, Bill Rodgers and Alberto Salazar made running go boom.* New York: Houghton Mifflin Harcourt.

Strecker, E., Foster, E.B., Taylor, K., Bell, L., and Pascoe, D.D. 2007. The effect of caffeine and ingestion on tennis skill performance and hydration status. *Med Sci Sports Exerc* 39:S43.

Stuart, G.R., Hopkins, W.G., Cook, C., and Cairns, S.P. 2006. Multiple effects of caffeine on simulated high-intensity team sport performance. *Med Sci Sports Exerc* 37:1998-2005.

Tucker, M.A., Hargreaves, J.M., Clarke, J.C., Dale, D.L., and Blackwell, G.J. 2013. The effect of caffeine on maximal oxygen uptake and vertical jump performance in male basketball players. *J Strength Cond Res* 27:382-387.

Vanakoski, J., Kosunen, V., Merirrine, E., and Seppala, T. 1998. Creatine and caffeine in anaerobic and aerobic exercise: effects of physical performance and pharmacokinetic considerations. *Int J Clin Pharmacol Therapeutics* 36:258-263.

Vandenbogaerde, T.J., and Hopkins, W.G. 2010. Monitoring acute effects on athletic performance with mixed linear modeling. *Med Sci Sports Exerc* 42:1339-1344.

Van Nieuwenhoven, M.A., Brouns, F., and Kovacs, E.M.R. 2005. The effect of two sports drinks and water on GI complaints and performance during an 18-km run. *Int J Sports Med* 26:281-285.

Vergauwen, L., Brouns, F., and Hespel, P. 1998. Carbohydrate supplementation improves stroke performance in tennis. *Med Sci Sports Exerc* 30:1289-1295.

Warren, G.L., Park, N.D., Maresca, R.D., McKibans, K.I., and Millard-Stafford, M.L. 2010. Effect of caffeine ingestion on muscular strength and endurance: a meta-analysis. *Med Sci Sports Exerc* 42:1375-1387.

Wemple, R.D., Lamb, D.R., and McKeever, K.H. 1997. Caffeine vs. caffeine-free sports drinks: effects on urine production at rest and during prolonged exercise. *Int J Sports Med* 18:40-46.

Wiles, J.D., Bird, S.R., Hopkins, J., and Riley, M. 1992. Effect of caffeinated coffee on running speed, respiratory factors, blood lactate and perceived exertion during 1500-m treadmill running. *Brit J Sports Med* 26:116-120.

Wiles, J.D., Coleman, D., Tegerdine, M., and Swaine, I.L. 2006. The effects of caffeine ingestion on performance time, speed and power during a laboratory-based 1 km cycling time-trial. *J Sports Sci* 24:1165-1171.

Williams, A.D., Cribb, P.J., Cooke, M.B., and Hayes, A. 2008. The effect of ephedra and caffeine on maximal strength and power in resistance-trained athletes. J Strength Cond Res.22(2):464-70

# Chapter 6 Known Side Effects, Health Risks, and Cautions

Arab, L. 2010. Epidemiologic evidence on coffee and cancer. *Nutr Cancer* 62:271-283.

Arria, A.M., Calderia, K.M., Kasperski, S.J., Vincent, K.B., Griffiths, R.R., and O'Grady, K.E. 2011. Energy drink consumption and increased risk for alcohol dependence. *Alcohol Clin Exp Res* 35:365-375.

Attila, S., and Cakir, B. 2011. Energy-drink consumption in college students and associated factors. *Nutr* 27:316-322.

Bell, D.G., Jacobs, I., and Ellerington, K. 2001. Effect of caffeine and ephedrine ingestion on anaerobic exercise performance. *Med Sci Sports Exerc* 33:1399-1403.

Bell, D.G., Jacobs, I., McLellan, T.M., and Zamecnik, J. 2000. Reducing the dose of combined caffeine and ephedrine preserves the ergogenic effect. *Aviat, Space Environ, Med* 71:415-419.

Bell, D.G., Jacobs, I., and Zamecnik, J. 1998. Effects of caffeine, ephedrine and their combination on time to exhaustion during high intensity exercise. *Eur J Appl Physiol Occup Physiol* 77:427-433.

Bell, D.G., McLellan, T.M., and Sabiston, C.M. 2002. Effect of ingesting caffeine and ephedrine on 10-km run performance. *Med Sci Sports Exerc* 34:344-349.

Bernstein, G.A., Carroll, M.E., Crosby, R.D., Perwien, A.R., Go, F.S., and Benowitz, N.L. 1994. Caffeine effects on learning, performance and anxiety in normal school-age children. *J Am Acad Child Adolesc Psych* 33:407-415.

Bernstein, G.A., Carroll, M.E., Dean, N.W., and Crosby, R.D. 1998. Caffeine withdrawal in normal school-age children. *J Am Acad Child Adolesc Psych* 37:858-865.

Bigaard, A.X. 2010. Risks of energy drinks in youths. *Arch Pediatr* 17:1625-1631.

Bramstedt, K.A. 2007. Caffeine use by children: the quest for enhancement. *Subst Use Misuse* 42:1237-1251.

Canadian Centre for Drug-Free Sport. 1993. The national school survey on drugs and sport. Ottawa, Ontario: Author.

Carvalho, M., Carmo, H., Costa, V.M., Capela, J.P., Pontes, H., Remiao, F., Carvalho, F., and Bastos, M.D. 2012. Toxicity of amphetamines: an update. *Arch Toxicol.* 86(8):1167-231. E-pub.

Conen, D., Chiuve, S.E., Everett, B.M., Zhang, S.M., Buring, J.E., and Albert, C.M. 2010. Caffeine consumption and incident atrial fibrillation in women. *Am J Clin Nutr* 92:509-514.

Daniels, J.W., Mole, P.A., Shaffrath, J.D., and Stebbins, C.L. 1998. Effects of caffeine on blood pressure, heart rate, and forearm blood flow during dynamic leg exercise. *J Appl Physiol* 85:154-159.

Frishman, W.H., Del Vecchio, A., Sanal, S., and Ismail, A. 2003. Cardiovascular manifestations of substance abuse, part 2: alcohol, amphetamines, heroin, cannabis, and caffeine. *Heart Dis* 5:253-271.

Garriott, J.C., Simmons, L.M., Polkis, A., and Mackell, M.A. 1985. Five cases of fatal overdose from caffeine-containing look-alike drugs. *J Anal Toxicol* 9:141-143.

Graham, T.E., and Spriet, L.L. 1995. Metabolic, catecholamine, and exercise performance: responses to various doses of caffeine. *J Appl Physiol* 78:867-874.

Griffiths, R.R., and Mumford, G.K. 1995. Caffeine—a drug of abuse? In *Psychopharmacology: The fourth generation of progress*, eds. F.E. Bloom and D.J. Kupfer, pp. 1699-1713. New York: Raven Press.

Grobbee, D.E., Rimm, E.B., Giovannucci, E., Colditz, G., Stampfer, M., and Willett, W. 1990. Coffee, caffeine, and cardiovascular disease in men. *N Engl J Med* 323:1026-1032.

Halloran, J. 2010. We won the title by using No-Doz-Mason. *The Sunday Telegraph.* www.dailytelegraph.com.au/sport/nrl/we-won-the-title-by-using-no-doz-mason/story-e6frexnr-1225899431505

Happonen, P., Laara, E., Hiltunen, L., and Luukinen, H. 2008. Coffee consumption and mortality in a 14-year follow-up of an elderly northern Finnish population. *Br J Nutr* 99:1354-1361.

Holmgren, P., Norden-Pettersson, L., and Ahlner, J. 2004. Caffeine fatalities—four case reports. *Forensic Sci Int* 139:71-73.

Hughes, J.R., and Hale, K.L. 1998. Behavioral effects of caffeine and other methylxanthines on children. *Exp Clin Psychopharm* 6:87-95.

Huxley, R., Lee, C.M., Barzi, F., Timmermeister, L., Czernichow, S., Perkovic, V., Grobbee, D.E., Batty, D., and Woodward, M. 2009. Coffee, decaffeinated coffee, and tea consumption in relation to incident type 2 diabetes: a systematic review with meta-analysis. *Arch Intern Med* 169:2053-2063.

Kaduk, K. 2012. Josh Hamilton and Rangers blame star's vision problems on too much caffeine. *Big League Stew.* http://sports.yahoo.com/blogs/mlb-big-league-stew/josh-hamilton-rangers-blame-vision-problems-too-much-2b5150810--mlb.html

Karlson, E.W., Mandl, L.A., Aweh, G.N., and Grodstein, F. 2003. Coffee consumption and risk of rheumatoid arthritis. *Arthritis Rheum* 48:3055-3060.

Kerrigan, S., and Lindsey, T. 2005. Fatal caffeine overdose: two case reports. *Forensic Sci Int* 153:67-69.

Kinugawa, T., Kurita, T., Nohara, R., and Smith, M.L. 2011. A case of atrial tachycardia sensitive to increased caffeine intake. *Int Heart J* 52:398-400.

Klatsky, A.L., Hasan, A.S., Armstrong, M.A., Udaltsova, N., and Morton, C. 2011. Coffee, caffeine, and risk of hospitalization for arrhythmias. *Perm J* 15:19-25.

Leson, C.L., McGuiggan, M.A., and Bryson, S.M. 1988. Caffeine overdose in an adolescent male. *J Toxicol Clin Toxicol* 26:407-415.

Lopez-Garcia, E., Rodriguez-Artalejo, F., Li, T.Y., Mukamal, K.J., Hu, F.B., and van Dam, R.M. 2011. Coffee consumption and mortality in women with cardiovascular disease. *Am J Clin Nutr* 94:218-224.

Lopez-Garcia, E., van Dam, R.M., Li, T.Y., Rodriguez-Artalejo, F., and Hu, F.B. 2008. The relationship of coffee consumption with mortality. *Ann Intern Med* 148:904-914.

Malinauskas, B.M., Aeby, V.G., Overton, R.F., Carpenter-Aeby, T., and Barber-Heidal, K. 2007. A survey of energy drink consumption patterns among college students. *Nutr J* 6:35-42.

Mattioli, A.V., Farinetti, A., Miloro, C., Pedrazzi, P., and Mattioli, G. 2011. Influence of coffee and caffeine consumption on atrial fibrillation in hypertensive patients. *Nutr Metab Cardiovasc Dis* 21:412-427.

McGee, M.B. 1980. Caffeine poisoning in a 19-year-old female. *J Forensic Sci* 25:29-32.

Mrvos, R.M., Reilly, P.E., Dean, B.S., and Krenzelok, E.P. 1989. Massive caffeine ingestion resulting in death. *Vet Hum Toxicol* 31:571-572.

Myers, M.G., and Basinski, A. 1992. Coffee and coronary heart disease. *Ach Int Med* 152:1767-1772.

Nawroot, P., Jordan, S., Eastwood, J., Rotstein, J., Hugenholtz, A., and Feeley, M. 2003. Effects of caffeine on human health. *Food Addit Contam* 20:1-30.

Nkondjock, A. 2009. Coffee consumption and the risk of cancer: an overview. *Cancer Lett* 277:121-125.

Norager, C.B., Jensen, N.B., Madsen, M.R., and Laurberg, S. 2005. Caffeine improves endurance in 75-year-old citizens: A randomized, double-blind, placebo-controlled crossover study. *J Appl Physiol* 99:2302-2306.

Norager, C.B., Jensen, N.B., Weimann, A., and Madsen, M.R. 2006. Metabolic effects of caffeine ingestion and physical work in 75-year-old citizens. A randomized, double-blind, placebo-controlled crossover study. *Clin Endocrinol* 65:223-228.

Nordt, S.P., Vilke, G.M., Clark, R.F., Lee Cantrell, F., Chan, T.C., Galinato, M., Nguyen, V., and Castillo, E.M. 2012. Energy drink use and adverse effects among emergency department patients. *J Community Health* 37:976-981.

Pacheco, A.H., Barreiros, N.S., Santos, I.S., and Kac, G. 2007. Caffeine consumption during preganacy and prevalence of low birth weight and prematurity; a systematic review. *Cad Saude Publica* 23:2897-2819.

Paganini-Hill, A., Kawas, C.H., and Corrada, M.M. (2007) Non-alcoholic beverage and caffeine consumption and mortality: the Leisure World Cohort Study. *Prev Med* 44:305-310.

Pasman, W.J., van Baak, M.A., Jeukendrup, A.E., and de Haan, A. 1995. The effect of different dosages of caffeine on endurance performance time. *Int J Sports Med* 16:225-230.

Peck, J.D., Leviton, A., and Cowan, L.D. 2010. A review of the epidemiologic evidence concerning the reproductive health effects of caffeine consumption: a 2000-2009 update. *Food Chem Toxicol* 48:2549-2576.

Pelchovitz, D.J., and Goldberger, J.J. 2011. Caffeine and cardiac arrhythmias: a review of the evidence. *Am J Med* 124:284-289.

Reis, J.P., Loria, C.M., Steffen, L.M., Zhou, X., van Horn, L., Siscovick, D.S., Jacobs, D.R., and Carr, J.J. 2010. Coffee, decaffeinated coffee, caffeine, and tea consumption in young adulthood and atherosclerosis later in life: the CARDIA study. *Arterioscler Thromb Vasc Biol* 30:2059-2066.

Reissig, C.J., Strain, E.C., and Griffiths, R.R. 2009. Caffeinated-energy drinks—a growing problem. *Drug Alcohol Depend* 99:1-10.

Ruhl, C.E., and Everhart, J.E. 2005. Coffee and tea consumption are associated with a lower incidence of chronic liver disease in the United States. *Gastroenterology* 129:1928-1936.

Shekellr, P.G., Hardy, M.L., Morton, S.C., Maglione, M., Mojica, W.A., Suttorp, M.J., Rhodes, S.L., Jungvig, L., and Gagne, J. 2003. Efficacy and safety of ephedra and ephedrine for weight loss and athletic performance: a meta-analysis. *J Am Med Assoc* 26:1537-1545.

Silverman, K., Evans, S.M., Strain, E.C., and Griffiths, R.R. 1992. Withdrawal syndrome after the double-blind cessation of caffeine consumption. *N Engl J Med* 327:1109-1114.

Snyder, S.H. 1984. Adenosine as a mediator of the behavioral effects of xanthines. 1984. In *Caffeine*, ed. P.B. Dews, pp. 129-141. Berlin: Springer-Verlag.

Spiller, G.A. 1998. *Caffeine*. New York: CRC Press.

Strain, E.C., Mumford, G.K., Silverman, K., and Griffiths, R.R. 1994. Caffeine dependence syndrome: evidence from case histories and experimental evaluations. *J Am Med Assoc* 272:1043-1048.

Tunnicliffe, J.M., and Shearer, J. 2008. Coffee, glucose homeostasis, and insulin resistance: physiological mechanisms and mediators. *Appl Physiol Nutr Met* 33:1290-1300.

Van Dam, R.M. 2008. Coffee consumption and risk of type II diabetes, cardiovascular diseases and cancer. *Appl Physiol Nutr Met* 33:1269-1283.

Van Dam, R.M., and Hu, F.B. 2005. Coffee consumption and risk of type II diabetes: A systematic review. *J Am Med Assoc* 294:97-104.

Vianni, R. 1993. The consumption of coffee. In *Caffeine, Coffee and Health*, ed. S. Garratini, pp. 17-42. New York: Raven Press.

Verster, J.C., Aufricht, C., and Alford, C. 2012. Energy drinks mixed with alcohol: misconceptions, myths, and facts. *Int J Gen Med* 5:187-198.

Winek, C.L., Wahba, W., Williams, K., Blenko, J., and Janssen, J. 1985. Caffeine fatality: a case report. *Forensci Sci Int* 29:207-211.

Wolk, B.J., Ganetsky, M., and Babu, K.M. 2012. Toxicity of energy drinks. *Curr Opin Pediatr* 24:243-251.

Zhang, W.L., Lopez-Garcia, E., Li, T.Y., Hu, F.B., and van Dam, R.M. 2009. Coffee consumption and risk of cardiovascular events and all-cause mortality among women with type 2 diabetes. 52:810-817.

# Chapter 7 Permissibility of Caffeine Use in Sport

Delbeke, F.T., and Debackere, M. 1984. Caffeine: use and abuse in sports. *Int J Sports Med* 5:179-182.

Del Coso, J., Muñoz, G., and Muñoz-Guerra, J. 2011 Prevalence of caffeine use in elite athletes following its removal from the World Anti-Doping Agency list of banned substances. *Appl Physiol Nutr Metab* 36:555-561.

López, J. 2010. Three-time champs lose title. *Nevada Sagebrush.* http://nevadasagebrush. com/blog/2010/03/02/three-time-champs-lose-title

Van Thuyne, W., and Delbeke, F.T. 2006. Distribution of caffeine levels in sport. *Int J Sports Med* 27:745-750.

Van Thuyne, W., Roels, K., and Delbeke, F.T. 2005. Distribution of caffeine levels in urine in different sports in relation to doping control. *Int J Sports Med* 9:714-718.

WADA Anti-Doping Code. 2012. List of Prohibited Substances and Methods. www.wada-ama. org/Documents/World_Anti-Doping_Program/WADP-Prohibited-list/2012/WADA_Prohibited_List_2012_EN.pdf.

WADA position on caffeine in sport. 2011. www.wada-ama.org/en/Science-Medicine/Prohibited-List/QA-on-2011-Prohibited-List.

WADA position on caffeine in sport. 2012. www.wada-ama.org/en/Science-Medicine/Prohibited-List/QA-on-2012-Prohibited-List.

# Chapter 8 Recovery and Other Considerations

Armstrong, L.E. 2002. Caffeine, body fluid–electrolyte balance, and exercise performance. *Int J Sport Nutr Exerc Metab* 12:189-206.

Armstrong, L.E., Pumerantz, A.C., Roti, M.W., Judelson, D.A., Watson, G., Dias, J.C., Sokmen, B., Casa, D.J., Maresh, C.M., Lieberman, H., and Kellogg, M. 2005. Fluid, electrolyte, and renal indices of hydration during 11 days of controlled caffeine consumption. *Int J Sport Nutr Exerc Metab* 15:252-265.

Beelen, M., Kranenburg, J., Senden, J.M., Kuipers, H., and Loon, L.J. 2012. Impact of caffeine and protein on postexercise muscle glycogen synthesis. *Med Sci Sports Exerc* 44:692-700.

Bonnet, M.H., and Arand, D.L.1992. Caffeine use as a model of acute and chronic insomnia. *Sleep* 15(6): 526-536.

Bryan, B., and Bryan, M. 2012. Waiting for Rafa and midnight Pringles. *The Age.* www.theage.com.au/sport/tennis/waiting-for-Rafa-and-midnight-Pringles-201220125-1qhsx.html

Cook, C., Beaven, C.M., Kilduff, L.P., and Drawer, S. 2012. Acute caffeine ingestion increases voluntarily chosen resistance training load following limited sleep. *Int J Sport Nutr Exerc Metab* 22(3): 157-164.

Ely, B.R., Ely, M.R., and Cheuvront, S.N. 2011. Marginal effects of a large caffeine dose on heat balance during exercise-heat stress. *Int J Sport Nutr Exerc Metab* 21:65-70.

Gregan, G. 2009. *Half back, half forward.* New York: MacMillan.

Maughan, R.J., and Griffin, J. 2003. Caffeine ingestion and fluid balance: a review. *J Hum Nutr Diet* 16:411-420.

Pedersen. D.J., Lessard, S.J., Coffey, V., Churchley, E.G., Wootton, A.M., Ng, T., Watt, M.J., and Hawley, J.A. 2008. High rates of muscle glycogen resynthesis after exhaustive exercise when carbohydrate is co-ingested with caffeine. *J Appl Physiol* 105:7-13.

Roehrs, T., and Roth, T. 2008. Caffeine: sleep and daytime sleepiness. *Sleep Med Rev* 12(2): 153-162.

Shea, B. 2012. 5-Hour Energy gets airtime as passenger on Mr. Furyk's wild ride at the U.S. Open. *For Immediate Release…* www.crainsdetroit.com/article/20120618/STAFFBLOG03/120619918/5-hour-energy-gets-airtime-as-passenger-on-mr-furyks-wild-ride-at-the-u-s-open#

Taylor, C., Higham, D., Close, G.L., and Morton, J.P. 2011. The effect of adding caffeine to postexercise carbohydrate feeding on subsequent high-intensity interval-running capacity compared with carbohydrate alone. *Int J Sport Nutr Exerc Metab* 21:410-406.

# Chapter 9 Individual Considerations for Caffeine Use

Ahrens, J.N., Lloyd, L.K., Crixell, S.H., and Walker, J.L. 2007. The effects of caffeine in women during aerobic-dance bench stepping. *Int J Sport Nutr Exerc Metab* 17:27-34.

Anderson, M.E., Bruce, C.R., Fraser, S.F., Stepto, N.K., Klein, R., Hopkins, W.G., and Hawley, J.A. 2000. Improved 2000-meter rowing performance in competitive oarswomen after caffeine ingestion. *Int J Sport Nutr Exerc Metab* 10:464-475.

Bangsbo, J., Jacobsen, K., Nordberg, N., Christensen, N.J., and Graham, T. 1992. Acute and habitual caffeine ingestion and metabolic responses to steady-state exercise. *J Appl Physiol* 72:1297-1303.

Bell, D.G., and McLellan, T.M. 2002. Exercise endurance 1, 3, and 6 h after caffeine ingestion in caffeine users and nonusers. *J Appl Physiol* 93:1227-1234.

Bell, D.G. and McLellan, T.M. 2003. Effect of repeated caffeine ingestion on repeated exhaustive exercise endurance. *Med Sci Sports Exerc* 35:1348-1354.

Bruce, C.R., Anderson, M.E., Fraser, S.F., Stepto, N.K., Klein, R., Hopkins, W.G., and Hawley, J.A. 2000. Enhancement of 2000-m rowing performance after caffeine ingestion. *Med Sci Sports Exerc* 32:1958-1963.

Carr, A.J., Gore, C.J., and Dawson, B. 2011. Induced alkalosis and caffeine supplementation: effects on 2,000-m rowing performance. *Int J Sport Nutr Exerc Metab* 21:357-364.

Conger, S.A., Warren, G.L., Hardy, M.A., and Millard-Stafford, M.L. 2011. Does caffeine added to carbohydrate provide additional ergogenic benefit for endurance? *Int J Sport Nutr Exerc Metab* 21:71-84.

Cornelis, M.C., El-Sohemy, A., and Campos, H. 2007. Genetic polymorphism of the adenosine A2A receptor is associated with habitual caffeine consumption. *Am J Clin Nutr* 86(1):240-4

Costill, D.L., Dalsky, G.P., and Fink, W.J. 1978. Effects of caffeine on metabolism and exercise performance. *Med Sci Sports* 10:155-158.

Cox, G.R., Desbrow, B., Montgomery, P.G., Anderson, M.E., Bruce, C.R., Macrides, T.A., Martin, D.T., Moquin, A., Roberts, A., Hawley, J.A., and Burke, L.M. 2002. Effect of different protocols of caffeine intake on metabolism and endurance performance. *J Appl Physiol* 93:990-999.

Doherty, M., Smith, P.M., Davison, R.C., and Hughes, M.G. 2002. Caffeine is ergogenic after supplementation of oral creatine monohydrate. *Med Sci Sports Exerc* 34:1785-1792.

Fisher, S.M., McMurray, R.G., Berry, M., Mar, M.H., and Forsythe, W.A. 1986. Influence of caffeine on exercise performance in habitual caffeine users. *Int J Sports Med* 7:276-280.

Flinn, S., Gregory, J., McNaughton, L.R., Tristram, S., and Davies, P. 1990. Caffeine ingestion prior to incremental cycling to exhaustion in recreational cyclists. *Int J Sports Med* 11:188-193.

Gliottoni, R.C., Meyers, J.R., Arngrimsson, S.A., Broglio, S.P., and Motl, R.W. 2009. Effect of caffeine on quadriceps muscle pain during acute cycling exercise in low versus high caffeine consumers. *Int J Sport Nutr Exerc Metab* 19:150-161.

Graham, T.E., Hibbert, E., and Sathasivam, P. 1998. Metabolic and exercise endurance effects of coffee and caffeine ingestion. *J Appl Physiol* 85:883-889.

Graham, T.E., and Spriet, L.L. 1991. Performance and metabolic responses to a high caffeine dose during prolonged exercise. *J Appl Physiol* 71:2292-2298.

Graham, T.E., and Spriet, L.L. 1995. Metabolic, catecholamine, and exercise performance: responses to various doses of caffeine. *J Appl Physiol* 78:867-874.

Hetzler, R.K., Warhaftig-Glynn, N., Thompson, D.L., Dowling, E., and Weltman, A. 1994. Effects of acute caffeine withdrawal on habituated male runners. *J Appl Physiol* 76:1043-1048.

Kamimori, G.H., Karyekar, C.S., Otterstetter, R., Cox, D.S., Balkin, T.J., and Belenky, G.L. 2002. The rate of absorption and relative bioavailability of caffeine administered in chewing gum vs. capsules to normal healthy volunteers. *Int J Pharm* 234:159-167.

Kilding, A.E., Overton, C., and Gleave, J. 2012. Effects of caffeine, sodium bicarbonate, and their combined ingestion on high-intensity cycling performance. *Int J Sport Nutr Exerc Metab* 22:175-183.

Kovacs, E.M.R., Stegen, J.H.S., and Brouns, F. 1998. Effect of caffeinated drinks on substrate metabolism, caffeine excretion, and performance. *J Appl Physiol* 85:709-715.

Lieberman, H.R. 2003. Nutrition, brain function and cognitive performance. *Appetite* 40:245-254.

McLean, C., and Graham, T.E. 2002. Effects of exercise and thermal stress on caffeine pharmacokinetics in men and eumenorrheic women. *J Appl Physiol* 93:1471-1478.

McLellan, T.M., and Bell, D.G. 2004. The impact of prior coffee consumption on the subsequent ergogenic effect of anhydrous caffeine. *Int J Sports Nutr Exerc Metab* 14:698-708.

Paton, C.D., Lowe, T., and Irvine, A. 2010. Caffeinated chewing gum increases repeated sprint performance and augments increases in testosterone in competitive cyclists. *Eur J Appl Physiol* 110:1243-1250.

Pruscino, C.L., Ross, M.L., Gregory, J.R., Savage, B., and Flanagan, T.R. 2008. The effects of sodium bicarbonate, caffeine and their combination on repeated 200-m freestyle performance. *Int J Sport Nutr Exerc Metab* 18:116-130.

Spriet, L.L., MacLean, D.A., Dyck, D.J., Hultman, E., Cederblad, G., and Graham, T.E. 1992. Caffeine ingestion and muscle metabolism during prolonged exercise in humans. *Am J Physiol* 262:E891-E898.

Vandenberghe, K., Gillis, N., Van Leemputte, M., Van Hecke, P., Vanstapel, F., and Hespel, P. 1996. Caffeine counteracts the ergogenic action of muscle creatine loading. *J Appl Physiol* 80:452-457.

VanSoeren, M.H., and Graham, T.E. 1998. Effect of caffeine on metabolism, exercise endurance, and catecholamine responses after withdrawal. *J Appl Physiol* 85:1493-1501.

VanSoeren, M.H., Sathasivam, P., Spriet, L.L., and Graham, T.E. 1993. Caffeine metabolism and epinephrine responses during exercise in users and non-users. *J Appl Physiol* 75:805-812.

Weir, J., Noakes, T.D., Myburgh, K., and Adams, B. 1987. A high carbohydrate diet negates the metabolic effect of caffeine during exercise. *Med Sci Sports Exerc* 19:100-105.

Wiles, J.D., Bird, S.R., Hopkins, J., and Riley, M. 1992. Effect of caffeinated coffee on running speed, respiratory factors, blood lactate and perceived exertion during 1500-m treadmill running. *Brit J Sports Med* 26:116-120.

# Chapter 10 Putting It All Together

Crawford, S. 2010. Caffeine critics need to take a chill pill. *Sunday Herald Sun*. www.heraldsun.com.au/afl/more-news/caffeine-critics-need-to-take-a-chill-pill/story-e6frf9jf-1225890284314

# Index

Note: Page numbers followed by an italicized *f* or *t* refer to the figure or table on that page, respectively.

# About the Authors

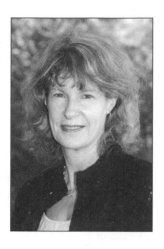

**Professor Louise Burke** is a sports dietician with nearly 30 years of experience in the counselling and education of elite athletes. Since 1990 she has served as the head of sports nutrition at the Australian Institute of Sport and served as the team dietician for the Australian Olympic team for five Summer Olympics from 1996-2012. Burke is also director of the International Olympic Committee diploma in sports nutrition and is part of the Nutrition Working Group of the IOC. Her research and education interests in sports supplements have included work on caffeine and sports performance.

Louise has a very modest caffeine habit. She hates coffee and has never tried an energy drink, and her daily caffeine intake consists (to her husband's annoyance) of half-cups of weak black tea. She is committed to practicing her (also very modest) sporting ability. Towards the end of her annual marathon she consumes caffeinated cola drinks or sports confectionary, which gets her to the finish line with a smile on her face.

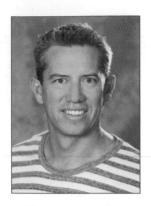

**Dr. Ben Desbrow** is a sports dietician and associate professor at Griffith University in Queensland, Australia. He completed his PhD in 2008 investigating the effects of cola beverages on endurance exercise performance. In 1999, Desbrow was awarded the first Nestlé Fellowship in Sports Nutrition at the Australian Institute of Sport. Since that time he has worked with many sporting groups, including the 2000 British Olympic team and the Australian Institute of Sport Cricket Centre of Excellence. Desbrow has co-authored numerous articles on caffeine use by both athletes and the general population for scientific nutrition journals. Desbrow is currently conducting new studies investigating caffeine's ability to influence exercise performance.

Ben has an addiction to iced coffee, which usually manifests as confusion around lunch time on most workdays. The solution can only be found by consuming 1 of 3 particular brands (he has a refined palate) or by his own homemade (secret) version. He completed his PhD investigating the effects of cola beverages on endurance performance--an achievement fuelled entirely by caffeine.

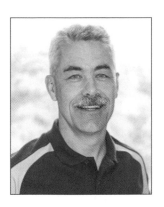

**Dr. Lawrence L. Spriet** is a professor in the department of human health and nutritional sciences at the University of Guelph in Guelph, Ontario, Canada. Dr Spriet received his bachelor's degree in kinesiology at the University of Waterloo, his master's degree in exercise physiology from York University in Toronto, and his doctoral degree in medical sciences from McMaster University. He was a post-doctoral fellow at Huddinge Hospital, Karolinska Institute in Stockholm, Sweden, and a visiting scientist in the School of Health Sciences, Deakin University, Melbourne, Australia. He has studied the regulation of fat and carbohydrate metabolism in skeletal muscle metabolism during exercise and has also worked on the effect of various nutritional and pharmacological interventions on athletic performance. His research output appears in numerous scientific journals, including Journal of Physiology, American Journal of Physiology, and Journal of Applied Physiology. Dr. Spriet is a member of the editorial board for the International Journal of Sports Medicine and the U.S.-based Sports Medicine Review Board of the Gatorade Sports Science Institute. He is also the chair of the Canadian Gatorade Sports Science Institute.

Lawrence is a committed caffeine user. He first sampled the benefits of coffee use while completing his MSc degree many years ago. Coffee now starts his every day, except when he's volunteering for a caffeine withdrawal study! Two to three additional cups of coffee punctuate the day, and just having the cup on the desk is a positive influence on the many tasks that need to be done.

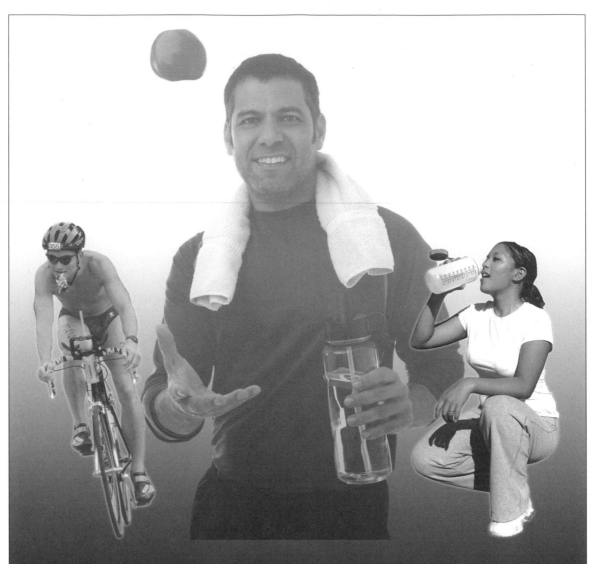

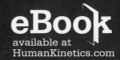